What Do the Readers Say?

When I announced on our free reader support forum that our book publisher wanted to include some FAT TO SKINNY reader stories in our new revised edition of *FTS*, many people wrote to me. They once stood where you are now, wondering if this little red book could be their answer to lifelong weight loss. They wrote to me, not because they are proud of their accomplishments (although I'm sure they are), but because they want to speak directly to you. These are people who feel your pain and understand your desire to finally lose your extra weight and become healthier. They, like me, know all too well the disappointment of yo-yo dieting and failed attempts at weight loss.

As you read the following pages, I want you to pretend that you're sitting in a room listening to stories from friends, because that's what these people will become to you. You'll meet them and have the opportunity to speak to them directly at the **FAT** TO SKINNY reader support forum. They will hold your hand and help guide you down the path to better health. Our reader forum is like a family and, as a family, we work together toward a common goal. You'll never be alone as you travel on your journey from **FAT** to SKINNY. The names you see above each story are the names these wonderful people use on our reader forum. Don't forget to say hello to them when you get the chance.

Be sure to visit and join the family at www.FATtoSKINNY.net.

Sherripie

Sherri lost 201 pounds in 15 months!

Taking Doug's advice, I cleaned out my pantry and logged on to the FAT TO SKINNY website. I posted my first post on the free reader support forum and declared I was going to change my life. I am proud to say, a year later and 201 pounds lost *forever*, that I am very glad I made that change. **I have gone from a size 32 to a size 14 in 15 months. That is more than *half* my size!** I still have a ways to go, but I have to tell you I am *thrilled* to be a size 14! I have made some amazing friends at FAT TO SKINNY, learned about eating correctly, and changed my life for the better. I want to thank all the forum members for listening to me complain, bitch, moan, threaten to bury the scale, laugh, and be amazed when it all works out. You are all great friends and I thank you for supporting me through this past year.

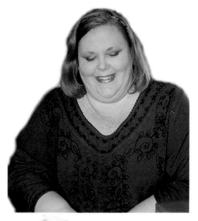

Follow Sherri's life-changing story at **www.FATtoSKINNY.net**.

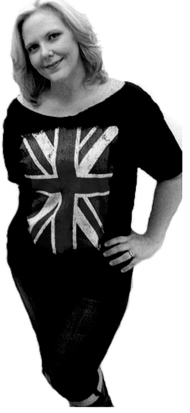

Gary lost 85 pounds in 8 months!

My name is Gary Koehler, and for a long time I was knocking on death's door. The years had taken their toll, and I had become **FAT** and lazy due to low energy, and also depressed. At 6'3", I was weighing in at 275 pounds with no relief in sight until April 12, 2010. That was the day my life changed. I was strolling through Barnes & Noble bookstore with my

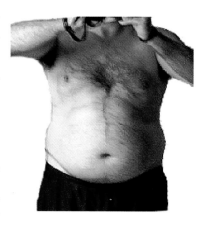

lovely wife when I happened across this bright yellow book titled *FAT TO SKINNY: Fast and Easy!* I picked it up, read through some pages, and said to myself, "I can do this!" Prior to this day I had tried many times to lose weight and get healthy, always to end up frustrated and still **FAT**. I even tried to convince myself that I didn't care, that I was happy being **FAT**, but deep inside I was still miserable. This is a picture I snapped of my gut the day I started *FAT TO SKINNY*.

I bought the book you're holding in your hands, and something inside me announced this time was going to be different. I read the book and joined the FAT TO SKINNY online support forum, where I found a family of people from all over who, like me, had discovered FAT TO SKINNY. This was a turning point in my life. With the support of Doug, his wife Sherri, and the encouragement from other forum members, I lost 85 pounds! It was amazing. I first set my goal weight at 200 pounds and, in less than 6 months, 75 pounds were gone forever and I had reached my goal. It was so easy, I reset my goal to 190 pounds and busted right through that to 188 pounds. ☺ This time was different; this time I succeeded! Here's a picture of my new and improved body 6 months after I started the program.

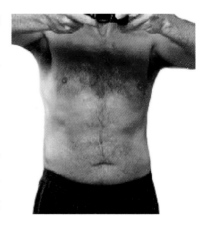

I'm no longer **FAT**, lazy, or depressed. I'm on FTS maintenance now and have maintained my weight very easily for almost 6 months. This is not a diet or a fad; it's a lifestyle change that I now live daily. The FTS eating plan is very enjoyable and easy to follow. Gaining weight is never an issue. If I find myself putting on a couple of pounds I simply adjust my sugar intake and BOOM, the weight drops right back off!

Before I started the FAT TO SKINNY program I was *squeezing* into 44"-waist pants. Today I am *very* comfortable in a size 34". ☺

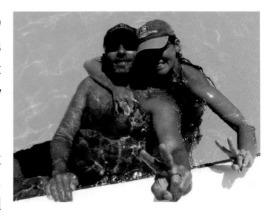

By picking up this book you've taken the first step. Now get busy and join me and countless others in finding the "skinny you" hidden within yourself. I look forward to meeting you on the FTS reader forum. Just look for Katary; I'll be there to help you through. Don't be a chicken—jump into FTS, the water's great! ☺

Follow Gary's life-changing story at **www.FATtoSKINNY.net**.

ShihTzuMom1

It took Patti 10 years to take off 17 pounds with conventional dieting and only 7 months to take off 41 pounds on FAT TO SKINNY!

I did it! I lost 58.5 pounds. ☺ Thank you, Doug, for writing *FAT TO SKINNY* and changing my life! I had been struggling for years: yo-yo dieting to take off weight, only to put it back on again. It has taken me 11 years to take off 58 pounds to reach my goal weight. The last 41 pounds of this weight loss (over a 7-month period) has been by

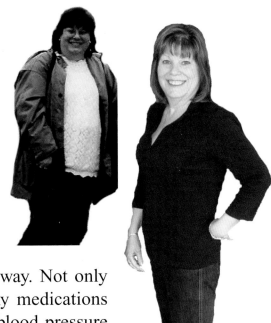

eating the FAT TO SKINNY way. Not only have I lost the weight, but my medications for type 2 diabetes and high blood pressure have been greatly reduced. I have found this way of eating so easy, without those nagging cravings, and also without the feeling that I am missing out on anything. I love that my favorite foods have not just been taken away, but have been replaced by something very similar. So again, I thank you, Doug, and your wife, Sherri, as well as the members of the FAT TO SKINNY online forum for all of your encouragement and suggestions to get me to where I am today. I seem to be doing well so far with maintaining my goal weight and feel that I will have no problem continuing with the FAT TO SKINNY lifestyle.

Follow Patti's life-changing story at www.FATtoSKINNY.net.

ScottinFlorida

Scott Johnson from Safety Harbor, Florida, lost 50 pounds in 6½ months!

I remember the day I was browsing in my local bookstore and saw *FAT TO SKINNY* on the shelf with this skinny guy on the cover holding up a pair of **FAT** pants. I'm so glad it caught my eye. After seeing my weight go up and down (more up than down), I was ready for a good long-term solution. I started this different way of eating a few days later and actually found it very easy. Twenty-six weeks later I had lost 50 pounds! While it is nice to feel great and be healthy again, one of the most wonderful results of this experience is I'm able to get back to something I really love—running! The interesting part about this is, running is not what enabled me to lose the weight. It was losing the weight that enabled me to run. It's still hard for me to believe: not long ago I was sedentary and overweight, and now I'm planning to run a marathon!

Follow Scott's life-changing story at www.FATtoSKINNY.net.

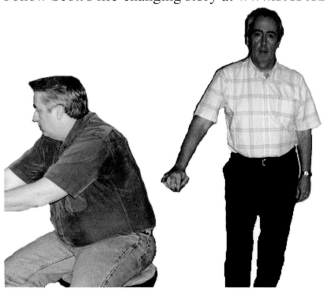

DoreenBar

She finally "gets it" for the first time in her life and melts off 62 pounds with no effort!

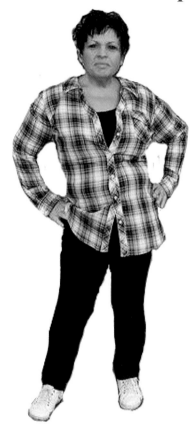

My name is Doreen, and if it wasn't for *FAT TO SKINNY: Fast and Easy!* by my wonderful friend Doug Varrieur I'd never be down 62 pounds in 10 months. It was the absolute easiest and most enjoyable year losing weight and gaining confidence and just plain being comfortable in my own skin. To be told I'm an inspiration simply gives me more happiness than anyone knows. I'm not on a diet. It's a lifestyle for me, now that I finally *got it*! Thanks!

Sincerely, Doreen

Follow Doreen's life-changing story at
www.FATtoSKINNY.net.

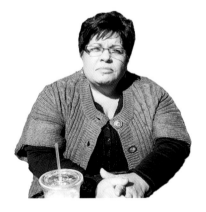

Izzet

"It still startles me when I see myself in a reflection or a mirror and I have to do a double-take!"

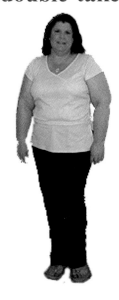

To my astonishment, in 6 months I went from a size 16 to a size 8, losing 36 pounds and lots of inches! My husband and I laugh when he says, "Where did you go?" I am full of energy and vitality and happy for the first time in years. Doug and Sherri (Doug's wife) take a very personal interest in your health, weight loss, and success. They are there to support you every step of the way on the reader forum with great recipe ideas, recipe conversions, and dealing with the issues that go along with weight loss. It still startles me when I see myself in a reflection or a mirror and I have to do a double-take. LOL I still can't believe it. Thanks to Doug and FAT TO SKINNY!

Follow Izzet's life-changing story at www.FATtoSKINNY.net.

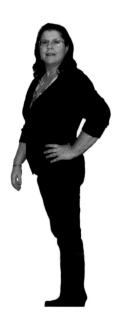

Richard

60-year-old man loses 52 pounds in 6 weeks, now feels like he's 30 again! Yes, *you can* change your life fast and easy with FAT TO SKINNY!

Doug, I thought I would let you know that since the second week in January I have lost 52 pounds. The thing that you didn't let me know is how much money I will be spending on new clothes. Even my shoes are getting too loose!

My doctor doesn't believe it either. I'll be 60 in June, and he's shocked that a person of my age has been able to shed all this weight so quickly without starving myself! He's scratching his head and now wants to do a complete blood profile on me.

Thanks, Doug, you are saving my life. And in the last three weeks I have gotten four other people on this lifestyle change. This weekend I worked on the farm like a 30-year-old. No joke—my wife had to stop me. Having a ball! Thanks! Richard

Follow Richard's life-changing story at www.FATtoSKINNY.net.

Mouseissue

59-year-old Tony reversed his diabetes, balanced his blood profile, and lost 54 pounds!

My name is Tony and I'm 59 years old. Before I started FAT TO SKINNY I was very overweight, had high blood pressure; a lousy blood profile, and I was a type 2 diabetic. I saw my doctor yesterday morning for my semiannual checkup, and got some good news . . . I've lost 54 pounds, my blood pressure is 106/72, and my doctor cut one of my high blood pressure medications in half. *Hooray!* By my next visit, he said that I may be free of all blood pressure medications if my weight continues to drop like it has up until now. Here are the stats:

Normal A1C (average plasma glucose concentration in the blood) level ranges from 4.5 to 6 percent. My A1C was 5.3 percent. My last reading was 6.8 percent. The doctor told me to stop taking Metformin for blood sugar control! **I'm no longer considered diabetic! Yippee!**

> Now for my blood results, they were excellent:
> Total Cholesterol 124
> LDL 66
> HDL 48
> Triglycerides 51
> FAT TO SKINNY is the bomb!

Follow Tony's life-changing story at www.FATtoSKINNY.net.

MaddysMom

Jan has lost her first 71 pounds, and she's well on her way to becoming thin and healthy!

Dear Mr. Varrieur,

Thank you so much for writing this book and sharing this life-changing information with everyone! I had struggled with weight problems and dieting most of my life. Your book made me realize that I didn't need a diet, I needed a lifestyle change. Though I have never had any serious medical conditions, I feel that I got my hands on this book just in time! I have lost a total of 71 pounds so far, and my personal physician is thrilled with my progress! I believe a big part of my success has been the support I have received from your free online forum at www.FATtoSKINNY.net. You, 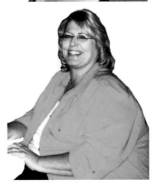 your beautiful wife Sherri, and all of the other wonderful people online have been so nice and helpful to answer all my questions! With the amazing recipes on the forum and in your cookbooks, I never feel deprived. I *love* being able to make cheesecakes, pancakes, and other great dishes . . . without the guilt!

I feel blessed that a friend cared enough to tell me about this book. Also, I am thankful that God has been faithful to bless my efforts as I continue on this path! Again, thank you! Enjoying the journey . . .

Jan Strickland, Gainesville, Georgia

Follow Jan's life-changing story at www.FATtoSKINNY.net.

Owensmath

Donna has lost 79 pounds and reversed her type 2 diabetes!

My name is Donna Owens, and here's my story. I had just been told by a doctor that I had type 2 diabetes and that I should eat a lot of lettuce, drink a lot of water, stay hungry all the time, and take these pills! I saw Doug on the *700 Club* one morning being interviewed about his book *FAT TO SKINNY,* and I felt it was divine intervention. I was depressed, hopeless, unhealthy, and morbidly obese. I read *FAT TO SKINNY,* joined the reader forum, and haven't looked back since. Before I began FTS my A1C (blood sugar reading) was 11, diabetic. Three months after starting FTS it had dropped to 6.4! My doctor couldn't believe it had dropped so far in such a short time. The next time I had my blood work done it was 5.8! I feel so much better than I have ever felt, I have more energy, and I have lost 79 pounds! Prior to FAT TO SKINNY I had tried all the diets and none of them ever worked. Living the FAT TO SKINNY lifestyle has been easy, enjoyable, and the best decision I have ever made.

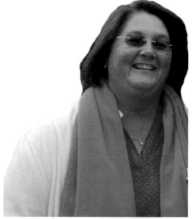

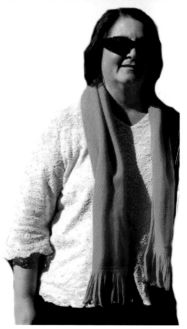

Follow Donna's life-changing story at **www.FATtoSKINNY.net**.

Rena

Rena has lost 53 pounds in 6 months!

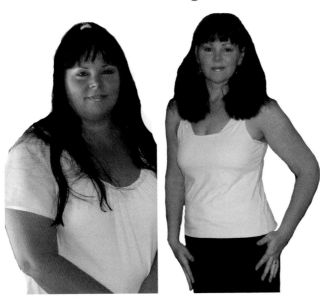

My husband bought the FAT TO SKINNY book and asked me to read it. I didn't want to because I was just trying to watch my portions. I read it reluctantly and decided to try the program for 1 month. In a period of 6 months I've lost 53 pounds and am still losing. In addition, I've been able to completely stop taking medicine for high blood pressure. I still have 21 more pounds I'd like to lose, but believe I can do it following the FTS program. Doug's book and the online forum have made losing weight *so* easy!

Follow Rena's life-changing story at www.FATtoSKINNY.net.

FAT TO SKINNY Fast and Easy! Revised and Expanded with Over 200 Recipes

Eat Great, Lose Weight, and Lower Blood Sugar without Exercise

Doug Varrieur

With recipe contributions from
Sherri Varrieur and Jennifer Varrieur

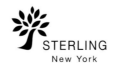

STERLING
New York

STERLING
New York

An Imprint of Sterling Publishing
387 Park Avenue South
New York, NY 10016

ISBN 978-1-4027-8817-8 (hardcover)

Distributed in Canada by Sterling Publishing
c/o Canadian Manda Group, 165 Dufferin Street
Toronto, Ontario, Canada M6K 3H6
Distributed in the United Kingdom by GMC Distribution Services
Castle Place, 166 High Street, Lewes, East Sussex, England BN7 1XU
Distributed in Australia by Capricorn Link (Australia) Pty. Ltd.
P.O. Box 704, Windsor, NSW 2756, Australia

For information about custom editions, special sales, and premium and corporate purchases, please contact
Sterling Special Sales at 800-805-5489 or specialsales@sterlingpublishing.com.

Manufactured in China

2 4 6 8 10 9 7 5 3 1

www.sterlingpublishing.com

This book is dedicated to all the

Special People

who simply want to be normal

HOW IT ALL BEGAN

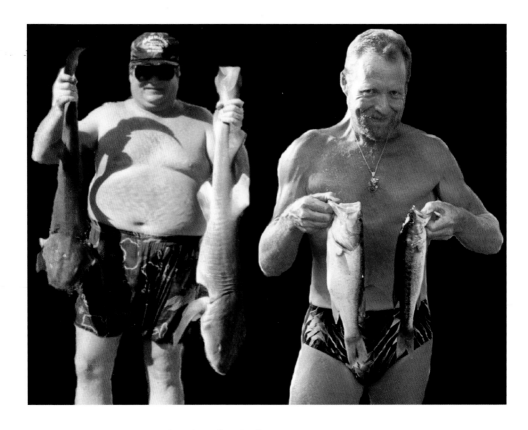

FAT TO SKINNY

Yes, this is me in both photos. In the **FAT** picture, I'm 35 years old and weigh 260 pounds. In the SKINNY picture I weigh 160 pounds and am 50 years old. At this point in my life, I've kept off the 100 pounds I *melted* away for many years. Want to know how? Read on!

In 2008 my book *FAT TO SKINNY: Fast and Easy!* was published and became a smashing success. Readers everywhere are losing weight, balancing their blood sugar, and finding a new lease on life from the information within its pages. I get thousands of e-mails from readers requesting more of the delicious recipes that make the FAT TO SKINNY program easy to follow and stay on. This was the inspiration for this follow-up book, the revised and updated *FAT TO SKINNY: Fast and Easy!*

Within the pages of this book you will find a delicious variety of low-sugar/low-carb meals to make your eating experience varied and exciting. You'll be amazed at the flavors you'll enjoy with quick easy recipes designed to satisfy your every urge.

CONTENTS

PREFACE

As a practicing family physician, I find that there is perhaps no subject of greater overall importance to my patients than obesity. Don't get me wrong—tobacco and alcohol use are right there, too, but neither of those is as rampant as obesity while crossing all age lines. I could bore you with statistics, but if you're reading this, I'll bet you're dealing with a weight issue yourself or have a friend, family member, or colleague with weight-related problems. If that's the case, please read on, because you're holding the answers in your hands.

For many of my patients, obesity has become the common denominator in the most prevalent diseases of our times. Obesity underlies all the big hitters, such as heart disease and diabetes, and it puts us at risk for cancer. It also leads to high blood pressure, high cholesterol, and high triglycerides, as well as the now famous "metabolic syndrome." It affects self-esteem, relationships, health, and job performance, and limits productivity. Yet as common as this problem is, most people have a poor understanding of its cause and feel totally helpless when it comes to dealing with excess weight. Is it any wonder? We have been bombarded with more bad information by businesses and experts than we can process. Some push low-fat products, some push magic weight-loss pills, some expensive prepackaged foods, some have expensive exercise equipment, and, I'm embarrassed to say, many from my own profession push surgery as the answer. As for the food industry, as a whole they will tell you whatever you want to hear if there's a buck in it for them. *But . . . is it really that complicated?*

From a medical prospective, I have known for years that the main culprit to our growing obesity problem is simply the amount of sugar and foods that metabolize into sugar within our diets. However, I would struggle with how to relay this information in the brief time I had with my patients. You see, sugar is sneaky, and isn't as obvious as the bowl on your table filled with white granules or little cubes. Just how to communicate this to my patients was perplexing, until one day about two years ago.

It was winter 2009, and I was at the bookstore with my daughter. We had some time to kill before picking up her younger sister from kindergarten. This is our special routine: we stop at the bookstore, and my little girl pleads for one of the cookies in the coffee shop. Most times I cave in and while she eats her cookie, I just wander about looking at books and CDs. I was strolling around and a bright red book cover caught my eye. As I picked up the book from the display table the name jumped out at me: **FAT TO SKINNY: Fast and Easy!** by Doug Varrieur. "Fast and Easy," I snickered to myself, but I opened it up and started to read. I always look at diet books to see what they are "selling," and I thought this one probably wouldn't be any different from the rest. I was running out of time and only read enough to pique my curiosity before I had to leave. The next day I returned to the store and started where I left off. I was surprised—no, I was shocked . . . this guy was making sense! I couldn't believe it: I had finally found the tool I needed to coach my patients. I immediately bought all the copies they had in the store and the next day I started giving them to my patients.

This book you're holding in your hands helped me be a better coach. I started focusing and honing my conversations. I started getting results or, rather, my patients started "getting it" and they got the results. I also trimmed a few pounds myself as I became more aware of the hidden sugar in my own diet. As Doug and I both say, "This isn't rocket science." It's simply the truth, well-spoken, outlining the cause and solution for obesity, high blood sugar, insulin resistance, metabolic syndrome, and adult-onset diabetes.

I've given a lot of thought to why Doug's approach works while many others fail in the long run. The best way I can put it is that he gives you the vision to actually see the problem that's been hiding in plain sight. It's not just the sugar you see that's making you fat, it's the sugar that doesn't look like sugar, and there's plenty of it in our diets, more than you can imagine. Doug points out in shocking detail just how much sugar fruits, high-starch vegetables, and grains yield in the end. I tell my patients, "You may not see sugar, but your body does." Our bodies eventually break down against the onslaught.

This is not your typical diet, which focuses on short-term weight loss, only to regain the pounds when you revert back to the same old dietary habits. FAT TO SKINNY teaches you to see the obvious—seeing what is there to be seen, seeing what's in plain sight—and, once the "glasses" are on, you'll have the tools and vision for lifelong success! And you'll lose the weight without exercise! Don't get me wrong, exercise is good for you and you should exercise under your doctor's care and advice, but it is not the key to weight loss. Unfortunately, people are misled (again) into thinking that they must exercise like crazy to lose weight. This I'm certain sells lots of exercise equipment and gym memberships. I'll probably catch flak for that statement, but it's true. Just as it's not the fat in your diet making you fat, it's not the exercise that can make you skinny!

This program is all about the type of food you put in your body and how the body metabolizes that food. It's about managing your choices and understanding why certain foods make you FAT and how to replace them with foods that will make you skinny. That's the magic of this bright red book. You won't go without, because there's a replacement for everything and—*yes*—it's Fast and Easy once you understand the secrets found within its pages.

I am proud to be able to contribute to Doug's efforts to enlighten people as to the true cause of weight gain, obesity, and all those nasty associated diseases. In many ways, what Doug is doing with his writings and support forum will make a bigger impact on the country's health than anything a doctor could dream of accomplishing. I am so pleased to have found a book that explains everything I have been telling my patients for years. Now I can talk briefly with patients and hand them this bright red book, knowing that what is put forth in the text is everything I believe.

This is a seminal work that awakens us to what is all around us but yet invisible. Like water to a fish we have been unable to see what has been in front of us all the time. Water? What water? I don't see any water! Sugar? What sugar? I don't see any sugar! Unfortunately, our bodies do see all the sugar and respond with obesity and "metabolic syndrome." This book is a must-read for anyone interested in taking their health to the next level.

Sincerely yours,

Dr. Paul Cump, D.O.
Johns Island, South Carolina

FOREWORD

Every day in my medical practice I confront obesity and its related complications. In fact these may be the biggest issues I face as a physician, for they can reach far beyond the waistline. Even mild obesity can cause imbalances in our bodies leading to high triglyceride counts, out-of-control cholesterol, insulin resistance, type 2 diabetes, and heart disease.

Obesity is an "equal opportunity" disease; it doesn't discriminate based on race, social status, income, or education. The truth is, we are all susceptible to its onslaught. Doug Varrieur is a case in point. At the tender age of 12, Doug personified the fat kid, squeezing into size 38 jeans. By age 17 he had earned the nickname "Porky," and by middle age Doug had developed type 2 diabetes and suffered a near-fatal heart attack. At age 43, he made a conscious decision to make it his life's work to discover the answers to weight gain and weight loss. Luckily for us, he hit on a solution that not only changed his life but *can change yours, too.* Doug discovered that a single ingredient—*hidden sugar*—was responsible for his seemingly irreversible weight gain. After making this breakthrough, Doug lost 100 pounds, reversed his insulin resistance, and reversed his type 2 diabetes. Years later, he's still trim, healthy, energized, and raring to help others make the same life-changing discovery.

The result of Doug's seemingly never-ending passion for getting out the word resulted in this book. In *FAT TO SKINNY: Fast and Easy!* Doug tells his own inspiring story and gives us some startling facts about the ingredient we all hate to love and can't always see: sugar. For instance, did you know that a medium order of fast-food French fries metabolizes into the glucose equivalent of eating about 15 teaspoons of table sugar? Or that 2 cups of raisin bran results in as much blood sugar as eating 20 teaspoons of table sugar?

Doug has really demystified the processes that cause us to gain weight, and makes it easy to understand how to lose and then control weight, type 2 diabetes, and insulin resistance. His approach is so simple and clear that anyone can follow his formula for success. The magic of his program is that it makes sense to everyone.

I've always thought that weight loss is very difficult and requires more discipline than most of us have. But after reading this book I think you will see it is really quite simple. And it's all backed by sound, scientific evidence. As a busy family physician, I have long searched for a down-to-earth practical guide to losing weight. This book is that guide: whether you want to lose 10 pounds or 100 pounds, it lays down the foundation for you and holds your hand on the journey to a healthier life. It empowers and educates you for a lifetime of healthy eating and living. For the first time in your life you will discover exactly why your weight has been a problem for you and what to do about it.

If you're a serial dieter who has jumped from one fad diet to the next— dropping pounds and clothing sizes only to watch your waistline balloon a few months later—Doug's simple, no-nonsense approach to losing weight and *keeping it off* represents real hope. If you can get hidden sugar out of your life you will not only get skinny "fast and easy," you will balance your blood sugar and reclaim your health and good spirits—without sacrificing great food or spending all your time at the gym. On Doug's eating plan you won't go hungry or feel deprived (the usual causes for falling off the wagon). Take a look at some of the delicious recipes and meal plans at the back of the book and say good-bye to the diet-starvation blues.

You've taken the first step by picking up this book. I'm sure you, like many of us, have tried diet after diet with little or no long-term success. The fact that you're holding this book in your hands tells me you have the desire to make changes in your life to lose weight and improve your health. Your desire, coupled with the power of this book, will give you the formula for lifelong success.

The key to weight loss and a healthier you begins with unveiling the truth about the ingredients that actually create fat and pack on pounds. In the pages that follow, you will clearly see what those ingredients are, how to avoid them, and how to replace them with healthy alternatives.

Human nature dictates that most people simply don't care how much you know until they know how much you care. I can attest to how much Doug Varrieur cares. If there was ever a man on a mission to help you lose weight and regain your health, it's this man. You will go from FAT TO SKINNY, and best of all you will do it with help from a friend, someone who has "been there, done that." Doug Varrieur is not only my patient, he is also an inspiration to everyone with whom he comes into contact. I can't emphasize enough what a service to society Doug has done by writing this book. I urge you to read it and follow the plan, for you too can go from *FAT TO SKINNY Fast and Easy!*

David Grant Mulholland, MD
Waynesville, North Carolina

INTRODUCTION

I used to be a big **FAT** guy. At a height of 5'8", I weighed 285 pounds and sported a 48-inch waist. Along with my weight came low energy, sore joints, insulin resistance, and type 2 diabetes. I shopped at the big-and-tall stores and found myself wearing XXXL shirts. By the time I was in my mid-40s, it seemed as though I had tried every diet known to mankind without success. It's not that I didn't want to lose weight—quite the contrary, I wanted to lose it very badly—I could just never find a program that worked for me.

New diets always began the same way. First I would get excited about the possibility of getting skinny, next came the realization that I had to exercise, and finally came the food plan, which usually consisted of rabbit food and canned shakes or expensive prepackaged stuff that tasted like cardboard. I hated exercise then as much as I do now, and being a chef I have a set of taste buds that are spoiled by good food. I was doomed before I began, but I always tried to give new diets my best shot. Unfortunately, I would ultimately fail and find myself in that place of depression only a person in my situation can understand. It would be short-lived, however, because my favorite meal would always cheer me back up and I would justify the failure by telling myself this diet simply wasn't for my type of body.

It wasn't until the doctor told me I needed to begin injections for my diabetes that I became really concerned about how the extra weight was affecting my overall health. For me, this was a turning point. I was aware of the complications diabetes could cause to my body, and, quite frankly, it scared me to death. I asked the doctor to explain to me what the injections were and what they would accomplish. He told me the additional insulin from the injections was necessary to control my high blood sugar. After some in-office instructions, he sent me home with my care package of needles and insulin to begin this new chapter in my life.

I sat at the kitchen table and stared long and hard at the future presented before me. I hate needles, really *hate* needles, and here they were sitting in front of me calling my name. I couldn't help but ask myself how I got to this point in my life. I went to bed that night really depressed and angry at myself. I had come to the conclusion that I had done this to myself and no one but me was to blame.

I woke up the next morning with two words ringing in my ears: "blood sugar." The reason the new medication and those wretched needles were now sitting in my fridge was due to high blood sugar, *my* high blood sugar. I decided to take the day off from work and research the causes and effects of high blood sugar. As page after page, article after article unfolded in front of me I found myself at the cellular level of the human body. I discovered that blood sugar fluctuations were simply the result of how our bodies metabolize the foods we eat and the beverages we drink. I found that glucose (blood sugar) is our main fuel that we burn each day to survive, and then I discovered a sinister side of glucose: what we do not burn we store as **FAT**! By the end of the day I was amazed by what I had discovered. High blood sugar was the singular cause of all my problems. The big fat gut, the sore joints, the insulin resistance, the diabetes, and the box of needles in my refrigerator! I immediately placed a call to my doctor. I had questions to ask.

I met with my doctor, and he agreed that if I could bring down my blood sugar naturally he would reconsider his latest course of action. I handed him back the package of needles and insulin and walked out of his office on a mission.

Seven months later I walked back into my doctor's office, and he was amazed. I had lost 100 pounds, reversed my insulin resistance, reversed my type 2 diabetes, and my energy level was through the roof. All blood sugar medications were stopped, and my blood profile was that of a 20-year-old. I was now wearing a 32-inch pant size, medium shirts, and I did it all without drugs, surgery, or exercise.

The following pages will reveal to you the secrets of losing weight forever and teach you how to get your health back on track fast and easy. This program works for everyone of all ages, male or female. It doesn't matter how much weight you want to lose—10 pounds or 200 pounds—you, too, can EAT GREAT and LOSE WEIGHT on the FAT TO SKINNY plan. This is not a diet; you'll never diet again for the rest of your life. This is a lifestyle change that removes all the foods and beverages that metabolize into excess glucose and swaps them with delicious replacements that won't make you **FAT**.

FAT TO SKINNY is a revolution with an impressive following of very successful readers. We even offer you wonderful free support at the FAT TO SKINNY reader forum located at **www.FATtoSKINNY.net**.

This wonderful book will change your life forever. If you're ready to start *your* mission, the next step is up to you.

—Doug

IN THE BEGINNING

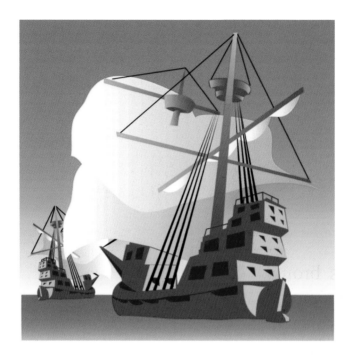

It all started with Columbus. You remember Columbus—everyone does. Columbus landed in the New World in 1492 and started the *maize craze*. Corn (maize) was a mainstay for the local Indians, and it wasn't long before this high-SUGAR, sweet-tasting vegetable was a big part of the diets of the colonists who followed. It was easy to grow and had lots of uses. Corn was used as a fresh vegetable, and as ground meal for bread, soups, puddings, and fried cakes. Corn was also used as currency by the settlers to trade for other essentials. The colonists also fed corn to their livestock to ***FATTEN*** them up. As a matter of fact, we're still feeding corn to our modern-day livestock to ***FATTEN*** them up.

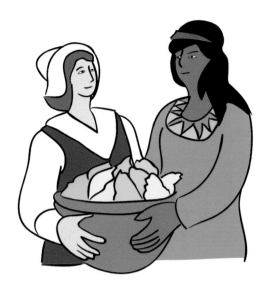

Columbus brought corn back to Spain, where it soon became an important food source across Europe. In 1493, Columbus brought a gift with him from the Canary Islands to the New World: *sugarcane*. Like corn, sugarcane also grows in tall, green, straight stalks. Once cut, the colonists would process it into SUGAR, which they used to sweeten their foods and beverages. They would then feed the pulp remains, along with corn, to their livestock. This was the beginning of the great American sweet tooth.

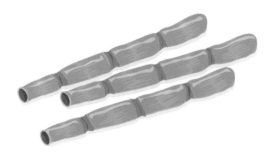

475 YEARS LATER

It was 1968, the country was heading into the Vietnam War, the Beatles had just released "Yellow Submarine," and Apollo 8 began its mission to the moon. I was 12 years old. Mom and I were at our local downtown clothing store. (This was before shopping malls were popular and small towns actually had downtown retail districts.) The store was called Joubert's and it was the town's only full-service clothing store. By full-service I mean the store catered to all sorts of folks' clothing needs, including the *special needs people*. There's a certain connotation to that label, *special needs people,* and at the tender age of 12, I was about to find out what it was.

After the tape measure and the calculations were complete, this was the day Mr. Joubert announced to Mom that I was a *special needs person.* Of course, at that age, I thought that was pretty cool. It was like being a part of an exclusive club…the Special Needs Club. My only question was, *What am I going to get for a prize?* I didn't have to wait long for my reward; it arrived in the form of a pair of **husky** jeans. Special jeans for *special people…husky jeans.* There weren't very many varieties of these special jeans available at Joubert's clothing store; I had a choice between blue or black. Mom bought both. On the way home, Mom explained to me that I was a husky guy, AKA a big-boned guy, and the *special* clothes for the *special* people cost more money, so I should take particular care of them. I guess she didn't trust my jean-care judgment, because as soon as we got home she ironed a set of leather knee patches onto my new husky jeans in preparation for my boyish abuse. In her wisdom, she decided I would ignore her advice and be as tough on my new huskies as I had always been on all my clothes. Of course, she was right, and before you could say husky, husky, husky, Mom had transformed my new Joubert's special person's pants right into something out of an old western. Unfortunately for me, it was just one more thing that made me different from the rest of the kids. At least I didn't have to wear kilts, like my younger brother David did. That's me on the left with my two brothers, David in the middle and Donald on the right.

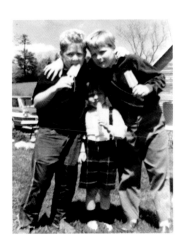

You're looking at a bona fide *special* person wearing bona fide *special* husky jeans while stuffing ice cream pops into his mouth.

Now, don't get me wrong—I knew I was fatter than the rest of the kids on my block. I was always the last one to get chosen for the backyard sports games, and wearing the most popular bathing suit of the day (Speedo) was completely out of the question. Mom always explained my size to me as being big-boned. "You'll grow out of it," she would tell me as she settled me down with…yes, you guessed it . . . food.

I'm not blaming Mom for anything, so don't misunderstand. Nutrition technology wasn't up to speed in those days, and most parents relied on the government's published food pyramid then as they do now as a baseline for their families' meal plans. Fast food really wasn't a part of the problem, because those types of restaurants were few and far between in our neck of the woods.

Over the next year, I grew, but I didn't grow out of "it" as Mom predicted, and I certainly wasn't in any shape to wear a *Speedo*. Instead, I grew out of my clothes as my waistline increased. By the time I was 13, I had ballooned to a size 38 pant. Mr. Joubert loved me—it was time for new huskies! That may not seem big by today's standards, but back when I was a kid childhood obesity was far less common than it is today. I was the **FAT** kid, and that was that.

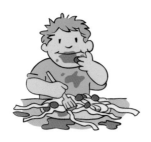

So there I was, the **FAT** kid, curly red hair, freckles, and with ridiculous patches on all my *special* pants. To make matters worse, I had to wear the wire headgear to straighten out my crooked teeth. All of this during school hours! YUCK! I'm amazed I survived childhood. There was no place for me in the social circles or on the school's sports teams. You know: *Fatty, fatty, 2 by 4, couldn't fit through the bathroom door*. Kids are cruel. I don't think most kids mean to be cruel; I think they mean to be popular, or cool. Cruelty is simply the byproduct. That is, until—as most kids do—I found my niche.

The Boy Scouts of America became my social circle (they know how to treat the *special* kids) and I prospered within that micro-society for the next couple of years. By age 15 I was sporting a 40-inch orb and, like lots of kids, struggling with teenage acne. The difference was I was the **FAT**, curly redheaded kid battling my new physical flaw: zits! At this point in my life, girls had not even been an interest, and considering them was out of the question. After all, who wants to go out with the pimply-faced **FAT** kid? No one I knew. Girls were, however, the initial motivation for this *special* big-boned kid to attempt his first diet. Girls and *Speedo* bathing suits.

I made an appointment to go to our family practitioner, Dr. MacEnroe. Dr. Mac was a no-nonsense doctor who seemed to always have an answer for everything bottled up in a syringe, so I was a tad nervous when I arrived at his office. Needles had always made me squeamish, and I was sure I was going to be stuck with one from his funny-looking black doctor's bag. Not the case, however; no needles that day. Instead, the good doctor told me I was in excess of 50 pounds overweight, and he prescribed me diet pills to curb my appetite and gave me a pre-printed diet plan to follow. He then sent me on my way with a watermelon lollipop in my mouth. And so it began, the dreaded diet. Even though it was 35 years ago, I remember it like it was yesterday. It all began with a helping of a diet pill followed by this eating plan:

Breakfast…Black coffee, dry toast, and a half grapefruit with no SUGAR on top.

Lunch…Water or juice, small green salad, scoop of tuna fish salad mixed with cottage cheese vs. mayo, and a package of saltines.

Dinner…Water or black coffee, 6 oz of meat or poultry or fish, small salad, and a piece of fruit.

The next day came, and it all began again and again and again! Some of you may remember the diet, or some variation of it. Of course, the problem with that diet is the difficulty of staying on it for any length of time due to its lack of variety and flavor. And let's not forget to mention the fact that the curly-headed **FAT** kid was walking around *speeding* his brains out from the diet pills! So, like many diets that followed, it failed, and I continued to struggle with my weight. What made matters worse was that my chosen profession was to be a cook. Talk about giving an addict an unlimited supply of food fix!

By age 17 I had fallen into my identity as the **FAT** guy and had adopted the nickname "Porky." This emblem was mine until I left high school.

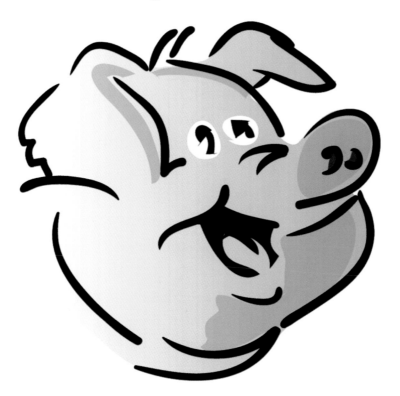

MY FIRST SUCCESS STORY

After I left high school, I took off and found my way to Texas. Having very little money and working two jobs, eating became a hit-and-run ordeal. I was busy, very busy, and I was motivated. My thoughts turned to straightening out my life and the food *issue* took a back seat. I ate less because I was running all the time. When I did eat, it was on the run, so I needed on-the-run food. I ate beef jerky, hard-boiled eggs, fruit, nuts, and veggies (such as celery sticks and bagged salads).

I was still living from paycheck to paycheck and restaurants were expensive, so I counted on a quick run into the local grocery store for food. When I wanted meat, I'd buy a small package of ham or turkey and a small block of cheese. Water was the beverage of the day because it was free. A simple stop at any public rest room filled my water bottle. This **FAT** guy found himself dropping weight like crazy and over the course of 6 months went from a 40-inch waist to a 32-inch waist. The first time I had ever been thin in my life! How simple…something else became more important to me than food! Without even realizing it, I had found a key, a key that I would later lose and not find again for over 25 years.

On my 18th birthday I called my mom to tell her about my weight loss and to bring her up to date on my life. I was proud to tell her I was no longer a *special person* at Joubert's and that I wasn't big-boned! Unfortunately, in my conversation with Mom, it became clear that I had to return home to handle some personal unfinished business that I should have handled before I left. It was time to say good-bye to Texas and head home.

Three weeks later, less than a year since I had left home, I arrived back in the little town of Whitman, MA. The **FAT** guy who had left returned home as the SKINNY guy. When I left, I had a big, bushy red afro, a 40-inch waist, and wore an army jacket with PORKY painted across the back. When I arrived home I was a 32-inch waist, had a clean haircut, and wore a suit and black patent leather shoes!

It was a glorious time for me. I settled into home life again and enjoyed living as a thin person for the first time in my life. Too bad it was short-lived.

MY FIRST FAILURE

In the first year after my homecoming, I went right back into the same eating habits I'd had prior to leaving. American Chop Suey was one of my favorite meals that Mom conjured up. The recipe calls for a pound of elbow macaroni, a can of Campbell's tomato soup, a large chopped onion, and ground beef. After the pasta is cooked, it is combined with the cooked meat, cooked onions, and soup to create Mom's delicacy. I loved it and always finished off a couple of bowls. Of course, it's Italian (sort of), so bread was a requirement with the meal.

Breakfasts were always fun and included fried potatoes at every sitting.

Lunch was typical: fluffernutter sandwiches, chips, and soda. For those of you who don't know what a fluffernutter sandwich is, it has peanut butter on one side of the bread and marshmallow fluff on the other. We also had strawberry fluff to shake it up a bit. Another favorite sandwich was banana and peanut butter. Just like ELVIS! It didn't take long for the weight to start coming back on.

My favorite vegetable was…you guessed it…corn! I loved corn, any way it came. On the cob, niblets, creamed—any way I could get it. Peas took a close second, and many times both were on the plate. Bread was served at every meal and I drank whole milk every day. My favorite snack was simply a banana, with a jar of peanut butter and a spoon to put it on top. Breakfast cereals—such as Fruit Loops and Cap'n Crunch—were always an arm's length away.

By age 20 I was **FAT** again. I never pieced together the food choices with my dramatic weight loss; I simply forgot. Food was so unimportant to me while I was in Texas that I simply credited the weight loss to all the exercise I was getting during my day job (walking in the Texas heat from home to home knocking doors) and to my night job (walking from station to station in the Levi's factory). I credited the weight loss to the lack of big, scheduled meals. The ingredient list was simply not focused on.

So there I was again, **FAT**. Not quite as **FAT** as before, but **FAT** all the same. My waist had ballooned back to a 38, and I struggled to keep it there. This struggle went on for the next 25 years. By age 30 I was bigger than ever. My waist was a size 44–46 and my weight hovered between 260 and 265. I was shopping in the Big and Tall stores and, once again, I had become a *special person.*

It was time to do something about it. It was time to focus on me. It was time to go on a serious diet. And so the battle began again…

THE **FAT**-FREE YEARS

Ah…the beginnings of yet another diet. This time I took the *fat-free* route. Fat-free products were all the rage, and I bought right into it. It was OK to eat potatoes—they're fat-free. It was OK to eat baked corn chips—they're fat-free. It was OK to eat peas and corn—they're fat-free. Fat-free salad dressings, fat-free mayonnaise, fat-free cheese, fat-free condiments, fat-free, fat-free, fat-free!

I lost weight. For me, the fat-free experience was responsible for the loss of about 30 pounds. Then… plateau. It didn't matter what I did; I couldn't drop another pound. For the next 13 years, the fat-free products helped my weight stay between 225 and 230 pounds. I had come to the realization that this was my "adult" weight, and if I could maintain it, I would be happy. I blamed it on metabolism, heritage, and age.

What I failed to blame it on was the one ingredient manufacturers of fat-free processed foods added back into their products. The ingredient to bring back the flavor they lost by removing the fat.

And then something magical happened.

FROM **FAT** TO SKINNY **AGAIN!**

Mom and Dad live next door to me in the Florida Keys. They come down for 5 months every year and arrive sometime in December. Their arrival on the year of my 43rd birthday was different from all the years prior. This was the year my Mom and Dad arrived and Mom was thin! I've failed to mention to you that Mom has also struggled with her weight over the years, and at the age of 71 she managed to lose 40 pounds over a 6-month period. I couldn't believe it when I saw her upon their arrival. She looked 20 years younger and had the energy level of a 40-year-old.

When I asked her how she lost all the weight, she answered with two words: SUGAR CONTROL! I didn't have a clue what she was talking about, so we sat and talked. She had gotten herself involved in a low-SUGAR diet at the recommendation of her diabetes doctor. She explained to me some of the foods her doctor warned her to stay away from. A lot of it didn't make sense to me, so I hopped onto the computer and started to learn. The information I found astounded me, and I found myself experiencing that old feeling of hope. I allowed myself to consider that I could once again be thin, just like I was for a brief period 25 years earlier in Texas. Maybe I'd even get thin enough to wear a Speedo bathing suit. I got serious about SUGAR, and what happened next was nothing short of a miracle… that all boiled down to simple biology.

WHAT HAPPENS TO YOUR FOOD AFTER YOU EAT IT?

In my research, I found that regardless of what you eat, all food breaks down into one of three groups:

PROTEINS

or

FATS

or

CARBOHYDRATES

CARBOHYDRATES then turn into SUGAR.

What I'm about to tell you is not difficult to understand. I'm not going to go on and on, page after page, about the chemical process. Instead, I'm going to explain it simply because it *is* simple. So simple, in fact, that even to this day, years after I shed that last 60 pounds, the weight stays off! If you follow the rules I'm about to lay out for you and understand the chemical process in your body, you too will drop all the unwanted **FAT** that you want to—and you'll keep it off!

Are you ready for the key?

If you constantly battle your weight and seem to have a predisposition to gain **FAT**, then you're consuming too much hidden SUGAR! And like most of us who constantly battle our weight, you just don't know it. You're also well on your way to becoming *insulin-resistant*, if you're not already there. We'll go into details about *insulin resistance* later in this book. The truth is, your weight gain and your inability to lose **FAT** is not your fault. (Unless, of course, you're a reader who is aware of your SUGAR intake and has ignored it. Then it *would* be your fault; you'd simply be lacking discipline, not knowledge.) I'll assume I'm surprising you right now and teaching you something you *don't* know. You're most likely addicted to SUGAR, like I am, and probably have been since a very young age.

Most overweight people crave and continue to eat foods they are addicted to day after day. We crave these foods because they make us *feel better* when we eat them. The average overweight or obese person has no idea that the daily food cravings and eating habits they are experiencing are the body's way of stopping *withdrawal symptoms* caused by the food addiction.

Why didn't Dr. Mac simply tell me I was addicted to SUGAR and high-SUGAR foods? The reason is that he— like most MDs and many other practitioners—simply wasn't aware of my addiction to SUGAR and its effects on my body. Only a specialist in this field would have been able to give me a diagnosis. Excess SUGAR and high-SUGAR foods in many people can—and does—cause weight gain and obesity, which in turn causes swelling, breathing problems, high blood pressure, heart danger, and in many cases, DEATH. The body's metabolic system simply can't keep up. The reaction to the body's inability to burn the daily intake of SUGAR results in excess **FAT**.

People's tolerance level to SUGAR will vary. In my case, I am a very active man, and still I am VERY sensitive to SUGAR in all forms. I gain weight very easily if my SUGAR intake exceeds 20 grams per day. Other people might not have such an intolerant disposition to SUGAR. Their metabolism may run more quickly than mine or yours, and they may be able to burn more of the high-glucose fuel with less effort. The easiest way to check your own tolerance is to remove SUGAR from your system altogether and start with a new baseline. That baseline will occur once you've attained your goal weight. At that point, you can experiment and start adding more SUGAR back into your system in measured amounts. These SUGARS will come in the form of *complex carbohydrates*.

SUGAR IS YOUR ENEMY!

SUGAR is what is making you **FAT**, and it's coming into your body from many different sources. Your body uses what it needs and then turns the rest into **FAT**. Once you know where all the SUGAR is coming from and understand what happens to it once it's in your body, you can start to make adjustments. Remember the gift of sugarcane from Columbus? It becomes *refined* SUGAR.

Refined SUGAR is found in processed foods, soda, candy, cookies, cake, ice cream, and any other products using it as an added ingredient. Refined SUGAR is a *simple carbohydrate.* The body burns it for fuel before it will burn anything else by immediately turning it into *glucose* (blood SUGAR).

SUGAR from fruits, *fructose,* is also a *simple carbo-hydrate.* Remember the body burns *simple carbohydrates* first for fuel before ever getting close to burning stored **FAT**. *Fructose* metabolizes more slowly because the liver converts it to *glycogen* prior to *glucose.*

SUGAR from vegetables and grains is a *complex carbohydrate* and burns more slowly than the simple carbohydrate. Although it burns more slowly, *excess* complex carbohydrates will also cause **FAT** gain.

Excess happens more quickly with grains than with vegetables. Grains get turned into flour, flour gets turned into breads and pasta, and bread and pasta break back down into SUGAR in your body. (I bet you eat lots of bread and other flour products, such as pasta.) Grains also get turned into cereal, and cereal breaks back down to SUGAR in your body. (I'll bet you eat a lot of cereal. You may even put a high-SUGAR fruit on top along with a teaspoonful of table SUGAR.)

SUGAR is going into your system at an alarming rate. It's in your vegetables, fruits, processed foods, snacks, condiments, beverages, breads, and flour. Americans *live* on SUGAR. I mean that literally when I say it. SUGARS and added SUGARS are the main fuel of the American public! According to U.S. Department of Agriculture (USDA) data, SUGAR consumption in 2005 was 142 pounds per person! And SUGAR consumption is on the rise. In 1983, each of us ate 113 pounds of the stuff. Our consumption has risen every year but two since 1983. The USDA surveys indicate that the 142-pound figure is equivalent to around 30 teaspoons of SUGAR per day! What is the result of all this SUGAR? Over the last 20 years in the U.S., we have seen a 100 percent increase in obesity rates in children and adolescents. Added SUGARS include regular table SUGAR derived from sugarcane and SUGAR beets (sucrose), corn syrup, high-fructose corn syrup, corn SUGAR (glucose), honey, and others. These figures do not include the SUGARS in milk, high-fructose fruits, grains, and high-sugar-content vegetables. All this SUGAR consumption over the years has created a vicious cycle for those of us addicted to SUGAR. The more SUGAR we eat, the more SUGAR we *crave.* Like the tobacco industry, it's the cravings that the SUGAR industry counts on to continue building its bottom-line profits.

So, now we know how much SUGAR we get from the SUGAR industry. How about the hidden SUGAR? This is the SUGAR coming into our bodies from high-SUGAR foods, such as fruits and vegetables. They come in the form of simple and complex carbohydrates. Four grams of carbohydrates metabolize the same as 4 grams of SUGAR. *To give you a visual, 4 grams of SUGAR equals 1 level teaspoon.*

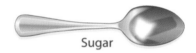

Sugar

So, how does our food compare to teaspoons of SUGAR? Let's analyze the SUGAR content in a medium order of fast-food French fries.

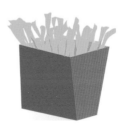

One of the purposes of your digestive tract is to break down the starch and other complex carbohydrates—which are simply chains of SUGAR molecules—into their component SUGARS so they can be absorbed into the blood. Our medium order of fries contains 47 grams of carbohydrates. Those 47 grams of carbohydrates metabolize the same as 47 grams of SUGAR, which is almost *12 teaspoons*! 12 teaspoons of SUGAR, just from the fries!

Now let's see what happens when we add a large soft drink, a hamburger bun, and a dessert:

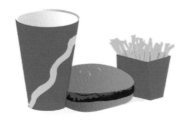
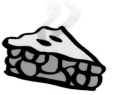

Sugar from fries	12 teaspoons
Sugar from soda	14 teaspoons
Sugar from bun	6 teaspoons
Sugar from peach pie	11 teaspoons

TOTAL SUGAR INTAKE: 43 teaspoons!

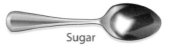

Imagine what happens to the counts when we "supersize" our orders. No wonder the obesity and type 2 diabetes problems in the U.S. are running at epidemic levels. Eating this lunch is the equivalent of sitting down in front of your SUGAR bowl and eating **43 teaspoons of SUGAR—almost 1 full cup!**

1 CUP holds 48 teaspoons.

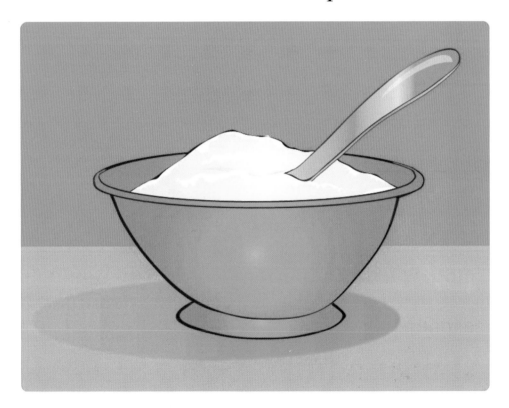

The only ingredient in the lunch that was SUGAR-free and good for you was the meat in the bun.

Now let's take a look at a typical breakfast.

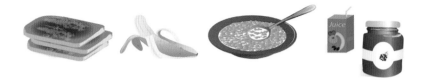

2 cups of corn flakes	**= 12 teaspoons of** SUGAR
1 normal size banana	**= 6 teaspoons of** SUGAR
2 pieces of toast	**= 8 teaspoons of** SUGAR
2 tablespoons of jelly	**= 7 teaspoons of** SUGAR
4 oz of milk on cereal	**= 1½ teaspoons of** SUGAR
6 oz box of orange juice	**= 5½ teaspoons of** SUGAR

TOTAL SUGAR INTAKE: 40 teaspoons!

Could you imagine how GROSS it would be to sit in front of your SUGAR bowl and eat 40 teaspoons of SUGAR?

Almost a full CUP of SUGAR

What about pizza? Pizza is one of our FAVORITE foods. There *can't* be any SUGAR in pizza…right?

Sorry! Let's take a look at a trip to the pizza parlor.

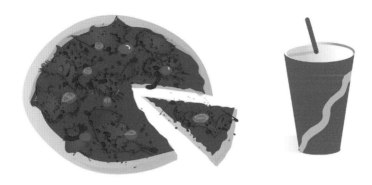

Pizza Hut 4-for-all Pizza Supreme

Whole pizza = **14½ teaspoons of** SUGAR

½ pizza for you = **7¼ teaspoons of** SUGAR

24 oz soda = **19 teaspoons of** SUGAR

TOTAL SUGAR INTAKE: 26¼ teaspoons!

If you ate that breakfast, that lunch, and then a Pizza Hut dinner, it would be the equivalent of eating **109 teaspoons of SUGAR. That's over 2¼ CUPS! So much for a healthy day of American eating!**

Now you see the problem with the American diet, and probably *your* diet. The problem is that our bodies are not burning all the food we eat, let alone our excess **FAT**. Our bodies are burning the crazy amount of SUGAR in our foods. The result is, all the SUGAR that doesn't get burned turns into what? You guessed it … more stored **FAT**!

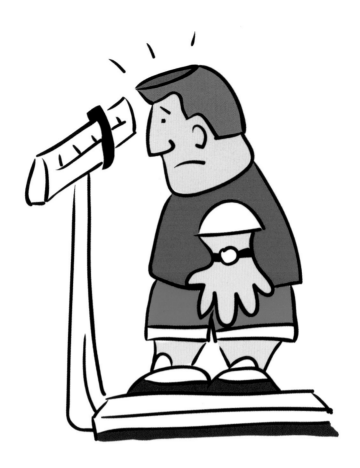

If you want to lose weight, your body needs to burn the stored SUGAR (**FAT**) for fuel. In order to get the body to do *that*, we simply have to cut off the SUGAR pipeline. This forces the body to attack those big, **FAT**, flabby deposits dangling around our bodies that make us the *special people* at Joubert's clothing store.

Cut off the SUGAR and you'll cut off the FAT. It's that simple.

So, how do we get rid of the SUGAR?

First we have to understand which foods in our diet are turning into SUGAR. Here's the answer: *all foods containing carbohydrates* turn into SUGAR… *gram for gram. 1 gram of carbohydrates = 1 gram of SUGAR. 4 grams of SUGAR = 1 teaspoon of SUGAR.* The body doesn't care what you eat or drink. It always breaks down the food or beverage into the same final ingredients. It doesn't matter whether the SUGAR begins as a complex carbohydrate SUGAR (found in flour and grains), a simple carbohydrate SUGAR (found in refined SUGAR additives), a fructose SUGAR (another simple carbohydrate SUGAR found in fruits), or a SUGAR derived from starch. All break down to the same thing—SUGAR—which in turn becomes glucose (blood SUGAR).

Carbohydrates In

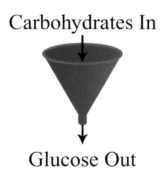

Glucose Out

Too much glucose, and BAM!! You get **FAT**, or worse, get **FAT** *and* develop **type 2 diabetes**. This disease is running rampant across our country, and you're at risk of developing it unless you curb the SUGAR. The following chart shows the SUGAR road.

All Roads Lead to SUGAR

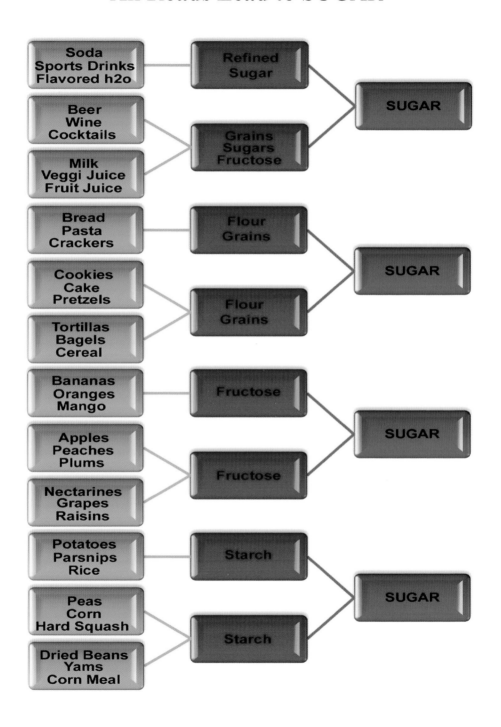

On the following pages I've outlined many common foods found in our diets. Next to each of the foods, I've broken down the SUGAR content in teaspoons. Take a look at this list and see how many of them are intermingled with your diet. Eating these foods gives you the same number of carbohydrates as if you were to eat the number of teaspoons of table SUGAR that I have listed beside each item.

From this point forward, I want you to **SEE** the hidden SUGARS in your food and imagine yourself sitting down at the SUGAR bowl with a teaspoon and eating pure SUGAR as you eat these foods. Then you'll see clearly the amount of SUGAR you consume daily.

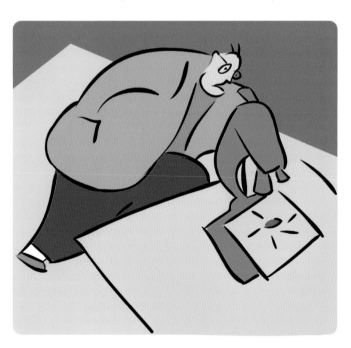

JUST A SPOONFUL OF SUGAR
HOW BAD CAN IT BE?

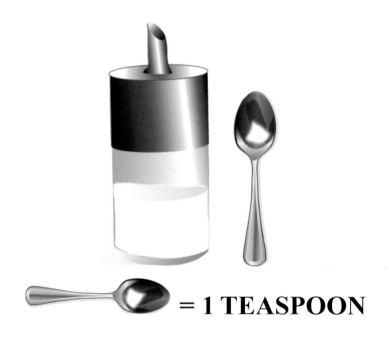

= 1 TEASPOON

48 = 1 cup

BEVERAGES

Soda (24 oz)	19	sugar
Orange juice (8 oz)	6½	sugar
Apple juice (8 oz)	7	sugar
Beer (12 oz)	3	sugar

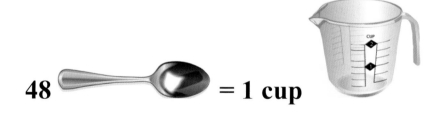

Milk 2% (8 oz)	3	sugar
Pina Colada (3½ oz)	6	sugar
Margarita (3½ oz)	3½	sugar
Hot chocolate (8 oz)	8	sugar
Gatorade (8 oz)	4	sugar

BREAD

I've eaten bread with every meal my whole life! Bagels were always one of my favorites until I discovered eating my bagel was the equivalent of eating 8 teaspoons of SUGAR right from the SUGAR bowl!

Bagel (3½ in)	8	sugar
Cornbread (5-in square)	9	sugar
English muffin, plain	6	sugar
English muffin, raisin	6½	sugar
French bread (3 oz)	9	sugar
Italian bread (3 oz)	9	sugar
Oatmeal (3 oz)	8	sugar
Pita, white (7 in)	7½	sugar
Pita, wheat (7 in)	7½	sugar
Pumpernickel (3 oz)	7½	sugar
Raisin bread (3 oz)	9	sugar
Rye bread (3 oz)	7½	sugar
Sourdough bread (3 oz)	9	sugar
Tortillas, corn, small	2½	sugar

Tortillas, flour, small	5½ 🥄	sugar
Tortillas, wheat, small	4 🥄	sugar
Tortilla, La Tortilla Factory	½ 🥄	sugar
Wheat bread (3 oz)	7½ 🥄	sugar
White bread (3 oz)	8½ 🥄	sugar
Whole grain bread (3 oz)	8 🥄	sugar

CEREALS

All 1-cup measurements

(I don't know about yours, but my cereal bowls all hold more than 1 cup!)

Cheerios	3½ 🥄	sugar
Cocoa Puffs	6½ 🥄	sugar
Corn Chex	6 🥄	sugar
Corn Flakes	6 🥄	sugar
Cracklin' Oat Bran	10 🥄	sugar
Cream of Wheat	7 🥄	sugar
Crispix	6 🥄	sugar
Fiber One	5 🥄	sugar
Frosted Flakes	9 🥄	sugar
Frosted Mini-Wheats	10 🥄	sugar
Froot Loops	7 🥄	sugar
Grape-Nuts	7 🥄	sugar

Grits	8	sugar
Life	8	sugar
Nut & Honey Crunch	7½	sugar
Puffed Rice	3	sugar
Raisin Bran	10	sugar
Rice Krispies	5½	sugar
Shredded Wheat	5	sugar
Special K	5½	sugar
Wheaties	5	sugar

CRACKERS

Cheez-It (20)	3	sugar
Harvest Crisps (20)	8½	sugar
Ritz (10)	5	sugar
Saltines (6)	3	sugar
Town House (8)	4	sugar
Triscuit (6)	4	sugar
Wheat Thins (20)	6	sugar

DESSERTS

Brownie (1)	6	sugar
Yellow cake (1/12)	9	sugar
Apple pie (1/8)	10	sugar
Cherry pie (1/8)	12	sugar

Milky Way (1 bar)	10	sugar
Hershey's Kisses (10)	7	sugar
Snickers (2 oz bar)	8	sugar
Oatmeal cookie (2)	8	sugar
Fig bar (4)	10	sugar

FRUITS

Apple	3½	sugar
Apricot (3)	2	sugar
Avocado, Haas	1	sugar
Banana (small)	4½	sugar
Blackberries (½ cup)	1	sugar
Blueberries (½ cup)	2½	sugar
Grapefruit	4	sugar
Grapes (1 cup)	7	sugar
Mango (1 cup)	6	sugar
Melon (1 cup)	4	sugar
Orange	3	sugar
Peach	2½	sugar
Pear	5	sugar
Pineapple (1 cup)	5	sugar
Raisins (½ cup)	13	sugar
Raspberries (½ cup)	1	sugar
Strawberries (½ cup)	½	sugar

PASTA & RICE

Pasta (1½ cups)	15	sugar
Pasta, wheat (1½ cups)	13	sugar
Rice, white (1 cup)	11	sugar
Rice, brown (1 cup)	11	sugar

SNACKS

Cheetos (30)	5	sugar
Fritos (30)	3	sugar
Pringles (20)	5	sugar
Pretzels (35 sticks)	4	sugar
Tortilla chips (30)	7½	sugar

By now you should have a good understanding of where your SUGAR is coming from. As you read labels, you'll look for the carbohydrate counts in the food. That's the way the FDA requires the food manufacturers to report the SUGAR content in our foods. Remember the formula: your body metabolizes every 4 grams of carbs the same as it would metabolize 1 teaspoon of SUGAR.

Remember the first diet I went on when I was fifteen? You know, the Dr. MacEnroe diet? Let's take a look at it again…this time we'll look at the numbers in terms of SUGAR content.

Breakfast…Black coffee, dry toast, and a half grapefruit, no SUGAR on top.

Lunch…Water or juice, small green salad, scoop of tuna fish salad mixed with cottage cheese vs. mayo, and a package of saltines.

Dinner…Water or black coffee, 6 oz of meat or poultry or fish, small salad, and a piece of fruit.

Let's examine Dr. MacEnroe's diet:

Black coffee	¼	sugar
Dry toast (2 pieces)	7	sugar
Half a grapefruit	4	sugar

Green salad	½	sugar
Tuna fish	0	sugar
Cottage cheese	½	sugar
Saltines (6)	3	sugar
Orange juice (8 oz)	5	sugar

Black coffee	¼	sugar
Meat (6 oz)	0	sugar
Green salad	½	sugar
Banana	4½	sugar

TOTAL SUGAR: 26 TEASPOONS! The equivalent of 104 grams of carbohydrates. We have to remove the fiber content from the carbs to get a **net** carb count. The fiber content for the day was only 6 grams. That leaves **98 grams** of **net** carbohydrates for Dr. Mac's daily diet! That equates into 98 grams of SUGAR divided by 4, which equals 24½ teaspoons of SUGAR!

If you're **FAT** and want to burn **FAT**, you need to keep your total intake to no more than **5 teaspoons of SUGAR from all sources per day.**

That means your total carbohydrate intake must be no more than **20 grams of total net carbohydrates for the entire day**. If you want your body to search out the **FAT** and use it for fuel, cut off the SUGAR fuel source by mouth and that's exactly what will happen. Your body will seek out the SUGAR it needs from the storage areas around your body. You'll shrink like the incredible shrinking person! And you can do it without being hungry.

No wonder Dr. Mac's diet and others like it have failed people for so many years. It's loaded with hidden SUGAR! This is also the problem with fat-free programs. Flavor is lost in products when they remove the **FAT**, so the manufacturers add another ingredient to make up for the flavor loss. Any guesses? I was amazed when I checked the labels. Most manufactures replace the **FAT** with…you guessed it…SUGAR! Again, the culprit in a **FAT**-free diet comes down to SUGAR.

I know what you're thinking. *He's taking away ALL my food. I have to starve myself.* Quite the contrary! If you follow this high-protein, low-SUGAR eating program, you'll never feel hungry. You'll eat wonderful food, and you will lose lots of **FAT** and keep it off! The trick is knowing what foods to eat, how to prepare them, and how to replace your favorite high-SUGAR foods with low-SUGAR foods.

I'm going to take all the guesswork out of it for you. As you continue to read on, you'll find I've outlined your new ingredient lists, given you favorite replacement recipes, and supplied you with Web links and products to keep your variety exciting. I'm also going to give you information about my blood profile and explain to you the effects on triglycerides and cholesterol that result from this kind of eating plan. In short, I'm going to dedicate the rest of this book to *you and your success* in the quest to be SKINNY. Your job is to understand the methods and apply them. *Knowing* the information is only half the battle; *doing something* with the information is the other half. One is no good without the other.

What do you say? Are you ready to get started on a new and slender you? Are you ready to fit into those high-school sizes again? Are you ready for your *miracle?*

Are You Ready to Slay the SUGAR Dragon?

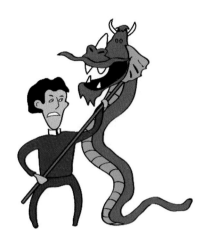

Let's Get Started!

First, we need to know how to read those labels. Let's take a look at this one. This is the pertinent information from the nutritional label for a 20-piece order of Chicken McNuggets from McDonald's:

NUTRITION FACTS
Serving size 20 pieces (320 grams)

Calories	840
Calories from Fat	441
Total Fat	49g
Saturated Fat	11g
Cholesterol	125mg
Sodium	2240mg
Total Carbohydrates	**51g**
Protein	50g

The ingredient you're looking for is
Total Carbohydrates   51 grams

51 grams divided by 4 equals 12¾ teaspoons of SUGAR. It will interest you to know that ALL of the SUGAR is coming from the coating on the chicken nuggets, and not from the chicken itself, nor from the oil used to cook it in.

The next product is chicken without a coating. Let's do another label. This one is the pertinent information from the nutritional label for frozen Tyson brand chicken breast strips. Let's look at the carb count in the chicken alone.

NUTRITION FACTS
Serving size 3 oz (84 grams)

Calories	120
Calories from Fat	32
Total Fat	3.5g
Saturated Fat	1g
Polyunsaturated Fat	.5g
Monounsaturated Fat	1.5g
Cholesterol	60mg
Sodium	500mg
Total Carbohydrates	**1g**
Protein	21g

Total Carbohydrates   1 gram

As you can see, the carb count in chicken without breading is VERY low. In this case, 1 gram per serving size, which is only ¼ teaspoon of SUGAR. That means you would have to eat 51 servings of this chicken to get the same amount of carbs into your body as you'll get from one 20-piece order of Chicken McNuggets!

Let's take a look at soda. This is a 14 oz mug of SUGAR-free A&W Root Beer. Here is the pertinent information from the nutritional label:

NUTRITION FACTS

Serving size 1 serving (397 grams)

Calories	0
Calories from Fat	0
Total Fat	0g
Sodium	35mg
Total Carbohydrates	**0g**
Protein	0g

Total Carbohydrates   0 grams

Below is another mug of root beer, 14 oz, and also A&W. Except, this mug is NOT SUGAR-free. This is the pertinent information from the nutritional label:

NUTRITION FACTS

Serving size 1 serving (397 grams)

Calories	190
Calories from Fat	0
Total Fat	0g
Sodium	35mg
Total Carbohydrates	**51g**
Sugars	**51g**
Protein	0g

Total Carbohydrates   51 grams

Look at the carbohydrate count: 51 grams. Now look at the SUGARS count. What do you see?…51 grams. Exactly the same as the carb count. The difference between the 2 sodas is the one that will make you **FAT** is the one that contains over 12 teaspoons of SUGAR (51 divided by 4 = 12¾). So what are we learning? It's ALL about choices. It's time to **LEARN YOUR FOOD!**

Now you know that an order of 20 Chicken McNuggets and a 14 oz mug of root beer contains over 63 teaspoons of SUGAR. You also now know that the same size serving of un-breaded chicken strips and a 14 oz mug of SUGAR-free root beer only contains ¼ teaspoon of SUGAR.

Which one are you going to eat? See, it's all about choices. Choose to eat products with VERY low carbohydrate counts on the labels and you'll lose **FAT**.

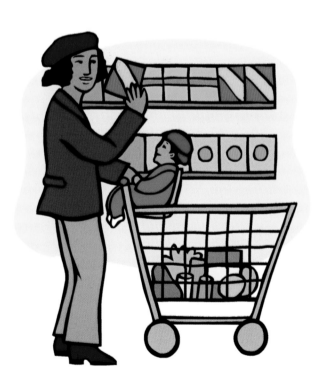

WHY DO I GET **FAT**?

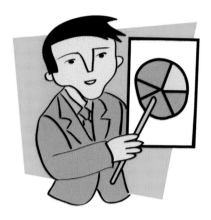

I know you're excited and more than ready to get this going, but we do need to touch on the science so you completely understand what is happening in your body. This is the stuff they should have taught us in grammar school! Let's start with proteins and fats. Both proteins and fats metabolize in your body slowly. They turn into fuel gradually, and they do not cause an *insulin reaction*. The only way you'll gain weight eating proteins and fats is by *over*eating proteins and fats.

Carbohydrates are completely different. Eating carbs does create an insulin reaction. It's that insulin reaction that causes weight gain. Here's the simple explanation: when you eat any high-glycemic (fancy word for SUGAR) foods high in carbs, the body turns it into *glucose*, AKA *blood SUGAR*, in your digestive tract. The glucose is then absorbed into your bloodstream. The SUGAR entering your bloodstream then causes the *pancreas* to pour insulin into the blood, creating an *insulin spike*.

Insulin is the ***gatekeeper*** for your cells. Each of your cells is a little ***furnace*** waiting for fuel to burn, but the fuel can't get in without the gatekeeper opening the gate. The job of insulin is to go to the cells floating around in your blood and attach itself to each cell. Once the insulin attaches itself to your cells, it opens up the cell to allow the SUGAR to enter the furnace to be burned. The body will burn what it needs based on your activity level, and then the *liver* converts all of the unused SUGAR into short- and long-term energy stores. Short-term glycogen is stored in your liver and muscle tissue, while long-term **FAT** gets stored in your **FAT** cells.

If you're **FAT**, it's because more SUGAR is going ***in*** than is being burned. Your chances of burning off more of the blood SUGAR increases dramatically if your body is revved up from strenuous exercise ***and*** you eat no more SUGAR than will burn off while your body is in a metabolizing state from that exercise. For most **FAT** people, that is not the case, but let's talk about *you*. When you sit down to eat a meal, are you within a half hour of coming from hard exercise? Or are you sitting at your desk, driving in your car, or watching TV?

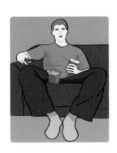

If you're like most of us **FAT** people, your body is sedentary when you eat and therefore has a less than fired-up metabolism. The furnaces in your cells are out. Your SUGAR intake is not getting burned; it's being stored for a rainy day inside your **FAT** cells. To make matters worse, you're probably into a bag of chips or snacks between meals, or worse, you ate a Big Mac in the car on the way home from work before dinner like I used to! All this SUGAR is causing insulin spikes.

It's the insulin spike that creates the problem. The insulin we produce in our bodies is our **FAT**-making hormone. Its job is to deal with the blood SUGAR by opening the furnace to allow it to be burned.

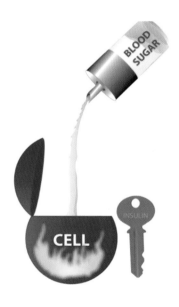

CELL
UNLOCKED BY INSULIN BURNING SUGAR

Once the body has burned all the fuel it needs, the fire in the furnace goes out. If you've taken in more SUGAR than the body needs, the liver will turn some of the excess glucose into glycogen for short-term energy stores, and the rest ends up in long-term storage as **FAT** to be reserved in your **FAT** cells.

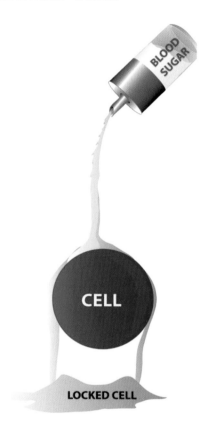

Locked Cell, Blood SUGAR Can't Get In

Fire's out, boys. Time to store the SUGAR!

Where do you guys want to stick it?

Let's put it in the **FAT** cells on the belly!

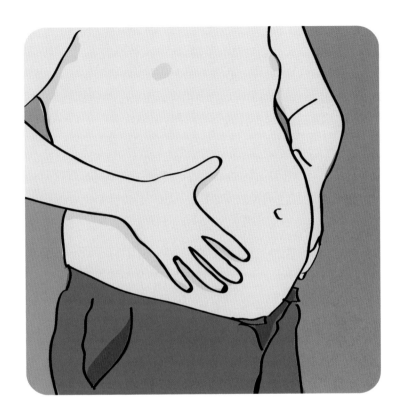

YOU CAN CHANGE THIS FAST AND EASY!

HOW DO I LOSE **FAT**?

Losing **FAT** is as simple as gaining **FAT**. To lose **FAT**, keep the SUGAR intake low and the glucose levels will stay low. Keep the glucose levels low and the insulin levels will stay low. Keep the insulin levels low and the **FAT** production ceases. It's that simple! All you need to do is switch fuels from fast-burning fuels (carbohydrates) to slow-burning fuels (proteins and fats). Your body will do the rest. Because of the enormity of the obesity problem in our country and the propaganda the diet industry feeds our minds, most of us believe the answer to **FAT** loss must be more complicated than this, but it's not. Fuel is fuel, and the body will seek out the fuel it needs within the body structure if you deny it entry by mouth. You don't need diet pills, you don't need expensive exercise equipment, you don't need to buy elixirs, and you don't need costly, prepared diet food shipped to your door. You simply have to understand body fuel.

This is the order in which your body burns fuel:

1st to burn, fuel #1—*Carbohydrates*, which have turned into glucose (blood SUGAR).

2nd to burn, fuel #2—*Glycogen*, stored glucose in the liver and muscle tissue.

3rd to burn, fuel #3—**FAT** *stores* in your body stored in **FAT** cells. The **FAT** you want to lose.

4th to burn, fuel #4—*Protein*, used to replenish body tissue. Any excess will be burned as fuel.

To get your body to the point where it starts burning your **FAT** stores, remove fuel #1, deplete fuel #2, and watch the magic begin.

To get your body to gain **FAT**, give it more SUGAR than can be burned during the corresponding insulin spike from eating excess fuel #1, and BINGO! You'll gain **FAT**. To get your body to stay the same weight and neither lose **FAT** nor gain **FAT**, only take in as much SUGAR from fuel #1 as you can burn during a particular activity. If all the SUGAR gets burned in the cells, you'll neither gain nor lose weight. It's all about scheduling your SUGAR intake based on:

Whether you want to lose **FAT**.

Whether you want to gain **FAT**.

Whether you want to stay the same weight.

Your goal should be to lose all the **FAT** you want until you get to the size you want to be. Once you're at your goal size, you'll want to maintain that size and not fluctuate more than 5 pounds either way for the rest of your life. You can maintain your new weight very simply by scheduling your food intake based on your activity level.

THIS IS NOT A DIET

This program is not a diet; it's the furthest thing from a diet. Diets don't work. The very thought of a diet leads us to the understanding that it is temporary. This eating plan is not temporary. This eating plan is an identification process of the one ingredient that has made you **FAT** and kept you **FAT**: SUGAR.

This is an opportunity that will train you to remove SUGAR from your everyday food intake, allowing you to live your life as a healthy, vibrant SKINNY person never fighting the weight battle again.

Knowledge is your hammer; SUGAR removal is your winning blow.

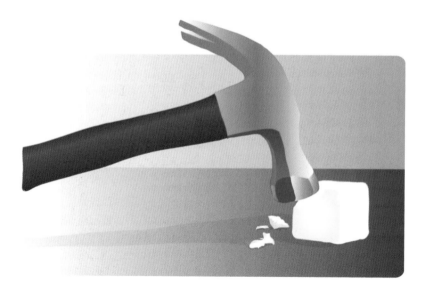

DEATH BY SUGAR

Now you know how your body metabolizes SUGAR, and you also know that the liver will turn unused SUGAR into **FAT** to be stored in your **FAT** cells. What if you don't make changes? What should you expect?

Overweight adults and children should be especially worried about their SUGAR intake. As we grow older, our metabolism slows, and the damage done by overeating SUGAR has taken a toll on our cells. Most overweight adults and many overweight children are already *insulin-resistant* and are well on their way to type 2 diabetes.

Insulin resistance occurs when the cells simply say "no" to the insulin trying to open the door to the furnace. The pancreas senses the high glucose level in the blood, and it sends out another surge of insulin to deal with the problem. Too much insulin can constrict your arteries and put you at risk for heart attacks. Excess insulin also stimulates your brain to make you hungry, creating the vicious cycle of SUGAR cravings. Of course, all the excess SUGAR stimulates your liver to manufacture **FAT**. As you grow older, all of this leads to high blood pressure, high blood triglyceride levels, and low levels of good HDL cholesterol. Next step for you? Type 2 diabetes.

Type 2 diabetes occurs once the cells quit responding to the insulin from your pancreas. Congratulations—you are now a diabetic! You have literally eaten yourself into diabetes. Diabetes leads to all sorts of nasty consequences, including (but not limited to) heart attacks, strokes, deafness, blindness, kidney failure, limb amputations, and DEATH.

Do I have your attention yet?

The good news is that all of this can be reversible, or at least substantially improved, by maintaining a low-SUGAR lifestyle. Several studies have shown that people may be able to eat their way out of insulin resistance and type 2 diabetes. In a June 2006 article, "Low Carb Diet Has Lasting Benefits in Obese Type 2 Diabetics," published by *Medscape Today*, a six-month study is reviewed in which two control groups, both overweight and both with type 2 diabetes, were observed. A control group ate a diet with substantially less SUGAR intake from carbohydrates than did the other group. Although the study was only six months long, the follow-up went on for 22 months. The conclusion of the study showed that after one year, patients with type 2 diabetes eating a low-SUGAR diet all had a lower number of hypoglycemic episodes, reduced glycated hemoglobin levels, reduced triglyceride levels, and stable levels of total cholesterol.

These conclusions are direct result of a low-carbohydrate diet and cannot be disputed. Cutting off SUGAR and foods that metabolize into SUGAR is a direct benefit on all fronts.

In another article, "Diabetes: America's Epidemic," written by Eileen M. Wright, M.D., Dr. Wright tells us that 2003 CDC statistics reveal that diabetes in the United States has increased by 61 percent since 1991! She reveals that an estimated 17 million Americans are diabetic, producing an annual cost of almost $92 billion! Of course this doesn't include the immeasurable cost of our national loss of lives due directly to SUGAR.

I liked her approach to it all; she agrees with me that one must "cut the head off the snake" by restricting SUGAR intake from foods containing carbohydrates like SUGAR soda, starchy vegetables, breads, rice, grains, desserts, cookies, candy, cereals and pasta to name a few, all of which can be labeled metabolic poisons for diabetics. In her article Dr. Wright advises the successful treatment for all diabetics begins with maintaining normal blood SUGAR. Of course, in order to maintain normal blood sugar, one must restrict the intake of high-SUGAR foods.

This is the basic principle behind the **Fat to Skinny** program. Medications to restrict blood sugar will never take the place of maintaining a healthy blood sugar level through diet and exercise. She concludes her article by agreeing with me that type 2 diabetes is reversible with simple diet and lifestyle changes. If you'd like to read her article, go to this Web address: **www.gsmcweb.com/?p=36**.

As you can see, it's up to you

LIFE

or

DEATH by SUGAR.

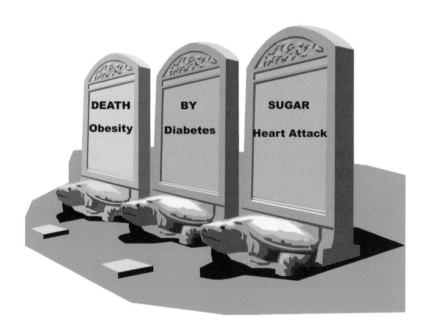

THE EXERCISE CONNECTION

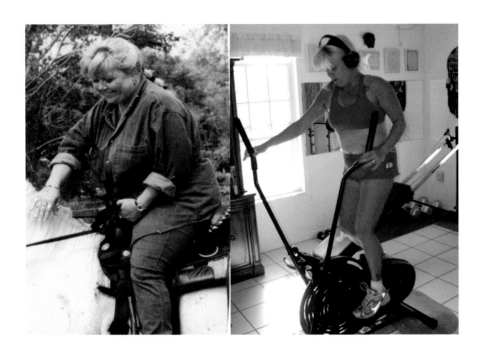

Don't exercise to lose weight! Eat **right** to lose weight. The above pictures are of my beautiful wife Sherri before a low-SUGAR eating plan, and then 70 pounds lighter after 6 months of low-SUGAR eating. She exercises for all the right reasons. She knows if you go into the gym or put on your jogging shoes to lose **FAT**, you're fighting an uphill battle. When you exercise to lose weight without changing your eating habits, you're simply battling your food intake.

Take, for example, our burger and medium order of fries. It takes 81 minutes of jogging at 5 mph to burn off the SUGAR derived from the hamburger bun and the fries! That's the wrong reason to be in the gym. You should exercise to build muscle, improve body tone, promote healthy circulatory and respiratory systems, increase your metabolism, and improve your attitude. Any weight loss you achieve from exercise is simply a bonus. Exercise does, however, increase the *speed* at which you'll lose **FAT** on this low-SUGAR program by increasing your metabolism. Your cells will require fuel from somewhere. Eating low-SUGAR forces the fuel to come from the stored **FAT**. Obviously, you would be far better off not eating the SUGAR to begin with. If you're eating the correct foods in balance with your everyday metabolism, you won't gain *any* **FAT** to burn off!

People who spend their lives working out to lose weight always end up **FAT** if they quit working out. Why? Because they don't change their eating habits. Here are some more examples of the amount of exercise required to simply burn off the SUGAR derived from the following foods:

25 minutes of aerobics for *each* pancake with syrup sitting in your pancake stack.

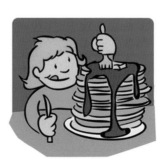

95 minutes of continuous swimming to burn off the SUGAR from an order of club sandwich and fries.

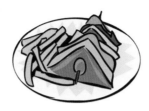

There is no SUGAR in the meat or the cheese, and there's very little in the veggies. The only SUGAR is coming from the bread and the fries.

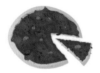

190 minutes of golf to burn off a personal pan pizza. There is no SUGAR in the cheese or the meat toppings. All of the SUGAR is coming from the pizza crust (and a few from the veggies and sauce).

It's all about choices. If you schedule your banana or your apple or your slice of pizza to coincide with an activity suited to burn off *all* the SUGAR intake, then that SUGAR won't turn into **FAT**. Once you've lost all the **FAT** you want, scheduled exercise will be a wonderful way to allow you to increase your carbohydrate intake without gaining **FAT**. Be careful of the trap, however. Most people can't stick to an exercise regimen long-term. If you rebuild your bad eating habits again by adding high-SUGAR foods back into your life and then quit working out, you'll get **FAT** again.

I don't worry about working out. I know that my everyday routine and my current SUGAR intake are in balance. For me, it's easier not to eat the bagel or the potato than it is to be forced into the gym by the food. *Always* eating low-SUGAR has allowed me the freedom to *choose* whether I want to work out on a particular day instead of being *forced* to work out by my SUGAR intake.

I know I'm a person who doesn't particularly like working out, and the gym comes in spurts for me. Usually, when I'm loaded with energy and stuck inside on a rainy day, my normal routine has me up and moving around. I'm doing something almost all the time. The only time I'm sedentary is in the evening or when I'm writing. You'll have to determine what kind of a person you are and whether exercise will play a part in your life. Some people are busy, but actually have less than physically active lifestyles; for example, the person who gets out of bed, drives to work, and sits, only to arrive back home by car to an easy chair. This is a person whose body has stayed fairly inactive all day long. This person needs to—at least—go for an evening stroll with the family pooch.

You need to be a realist. If you've failed up until now at keeping a scheduled exercise program in your life, then chances are you'll fail again. This is all the more reason NOT to put SUGAR into your body. I recommend exercise for all the right reasons, and fighting SUGAR intake in the gym isn't one of them. If you make the changes in your eating habits outlined in this book and eliminate SUGAR from your food intake, even the most sedentary person will lose **FAT**. If you're an active to very active person, you'll lose **FAT** faster. If you add some form of additional exercise into the mix, your weight loss will be even quicker. Simple arithmetic: the more fuel you burn, the faster the storage areas shrink. Exercise is *your* choice.

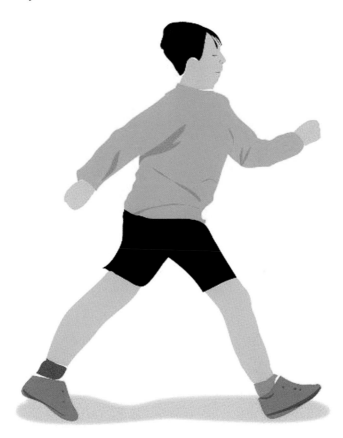

DON'T I NEED CARBOHYDRATES?

Yes, most definitely. Your brain and every one of your cells need carbohydrates to function properly. Modern science believes that the *average person* weighing in at a weight corresponding to their size and gender *and* maintaining a *"normal"* activity level needs upwards of 130 grams of carbohydrates a day for proper cell and brain function. Is that you?

Everyone is different. Numbers like those are based on averages. I certainly could not eat that level of SUGAR on a daily basis and maintain my current 32-inch waist! As mentioned earlier, my SUGAR intake needs to be kept at around 20 carbs per day. I am not sedentary; I live an active lifestyle, and you'll only occasionally see me in the gym. I consider myself of *normal* weight for my size: 165 pounds at 5'11". I also consider my activity level to be *normal*, so I don't fit into these guidelines. You probably don't, either, considering you're reading this book.

You'll have your chance to find out how much SUGAR you can eat once you've lost the **FAT**. Believe me, right now you have plenty of carbohydrates stored around your body that need to be burned before you start to replace them by mouth. Once you have become SKINNY by burning the **FAT** stores in your body, it will be important to start replacing your carbohydrates by mouth. The difference is you'll be giving your body the *best* carbohydrates by eating complex carbs found in whole grains and vegetables, plus simple carbs found in fruit, all of it in measured and controlled quantities. You'll know when you reach your personal metabolic threshold for SUGAR intake by keeping an eye on the scale. If your normal daily routine doesn't burn all the SUGAR you take in, you'll start to gain weight again. When that happens, you'll know you're above your threshold and you'll need to cut back until your body starts to lose weight again. Use your scale once a week in the morning, and keep track of your progress with a log.

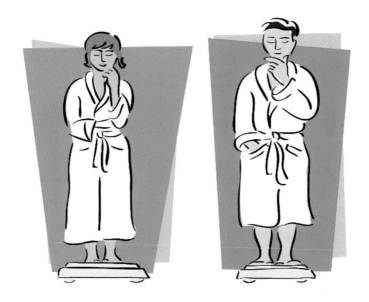

Make sure you keep a log and weigh yourself on a scheduled basis at the same time each week. This is especially important when you've lost all the weight you want. Ten pounds can come on quickly if you jump back into the SUGAR pipeline! The scale will keep you on your game.

SUGAR, THE GREAT BIG **FAT** LIE!

SUGAR is BIG business and does more than make us **FAT** around the midsection. SUGAR is responsible for many industries having **FAT** bottom lines! Christopher Columbus first introduced SUGAR to the New World at the end of the 15th century. By the 17th century, SUGAR production in the subtropical and tropical regions of the Americas had become the largest and most lucrative industry in the world. According to the U.S. Department of Commerce reports, SUGAR fuels (to name a few)…

Candy industry ($43 BILLION annual sales)

Soda pop industry ($70 BILLION in annual sales)

Snack industry ($57 BILLION in annual sales)

Diet industry ($35 BILLION in annual sales)

The International Sugar Journal reports, the U.S. SUGAR industry is one of the largest in the world, generating over 146,000 jobs. This industry is responsible for almost $10 BILLION in economic activity in the 19 states where sugar beets and sugarcane are grown and processed.

Now let's take a look at the economic impact of **type 2 diabetes**. According to the National Library of Medicine, costs to the nation are now approaching $20 billion. Not to mention the terrible toll it takes on the afflicted. And this is just the tip of the iceberg when it comes to how SUGAR-related diseases affect the medical industry. UNTOLD BILLIONS are spent annually by our population on afflictions which ultimately can be traced back to our insatiable addiction to SUGAR.

The facts seem undeniable: *economically*, our country is far better off if we are **FAT** and obese than it is if we are thin and slender. Our nation's SUGAR addiction fuels way too much business. I'm afraid you won't get any help from the government on this problem anytime soon, either; all you have to do is review the following **NEW** food pyramid proposed by the US government. I went to the government's food pyramid Web site. They have a page where I could enter my statistics and they would send me MY pyramid.

www.choosemyplate.gov/myplate/index.aspx

The Web site then calculated a "custom food pyramid" for me. It's LOADED with SUGAR! If I were to eat a diet relying on this information, I would be **FAT** as a cow in very short order and my SUGAR addiction would continue to be fueled. As you review my food pyramid, you'll notice the plan calls for me to consume the following foods on a weekly basis:

7 cups of grain	SUGAR
21 cups of high-carb veggies	SUGAR
14 cups of fruit	SUGAR

21 cups of low-fat milk	SUGAR
3 cups of beans, peas, nuts & seeds	SUGAR
5.5 cups of meat, fish or poultry	PROTEIN

It makes me wonder why the obvious and simplistic nutritional changes to lean out our nation are being completely ignored. Could it be economically driven? I'll leave that up to you to decide.

DOUG'S CUSTOM FOOD PYRAMID

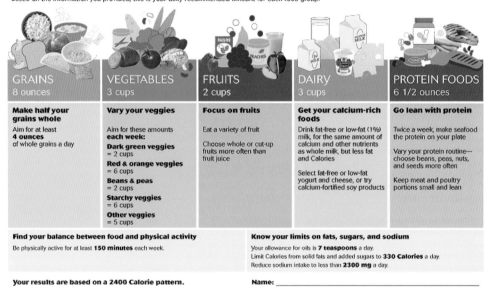

My Daily Food Plan

Based on the information you provided, this is your daily recommended amount for each food group.

GRAINS 8 ounces	VEGETABLES 3 cups	FRUITS 2 cups	DAIRY 3 cups	PROTEIN FOODS 6 1/2 ounces
Make half your grains whole	**Vary your veggies**	**Focus on fruits**	**Get your calcium-rich foods**	**Go lean with protein**
Aim for at least **4 ounces** of whole grains a day	Aim for these amounts each week: **Dark green veggies** = 2 cups **Red & orange veggies** = 6 cups **Beans & peas** = 2 cups **Starchy veggies** = 6 cups **Other veggies** = 5 cups	Eat a variety of fruit Choose whole or cut-up fruits more often than fruit juice	Drink fat-free or low-fat (1%) milk, for the same amount of calcium and other nutrients as whole milk, but less fat and Calories Select fat-free or low-fat yogurt and cheese, or try calcium-fortified soy products	Twice a week, make seafood the protein on your plate Vary your protein routine— choose beans, peas, nuts, and seeds more often Keep meat and poultry portions small and lean

Find your balance between food and physical activity
Be physically active for at least **150 minutes** each week.

Know your limits on fats, sugars, and sodium
Your allowance for oils is **7 teaspoons** a day.
Limit Calories from solid fats and added sugars to **330 Calories** a day.
Reduce sodium intake to less than **2300 mg** a day.

Your results are based on a 2400 Calorie pattern.   Name: _____

This Calorie level is only an estimate of your needs. Monitor your body weight to see if you need to adjust your Calorie intake.

Now let's compare my food pyramid to the diet of a meat steer. Is it possible people are eating COW FOOD? Author and small-scale cattleman Michael Pollan recently wrote about steer No. 534 in *The New York Times*. He followed No. 534 from birth to the slaughterhouse. In his article, entitled "Power Steer," he states that he fed No. 534 a daily diet of "14 pounds of corn and 6 pounds of hay—and added 2½ pounds every day to No. 534…On Nov. 13 he weighed 650 pounds; by Christmas he was up to 798…No. 534 put away 706 pounds of corn and 336 pounds of alfalfa hay." It's no secret that cow food is front-loaded with grains and corn to fatten up the cow for slaughter. After all, the rancher and everyone else get paid by the pound! GRAINS = SUGAR, SUGAR then turns into **FAT**. As I mentioned earlier, if I ate the diet plan outlined for me in my custom food pyramid, I would be as **FAT** as a COW! WHY? Because I would be eating COW FOOD. Cows eat corn and grains. Flour comes from ground GRAIN.

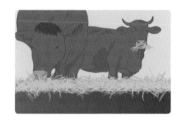 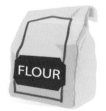

Flour is then processed into a zillion things, including bread, cookies, cake, bagels, tortillas, pasta, snacks, pretzels, etc., etc., etc. It's ALL cow food!

Ever notice how sleek and streamlined the great cats are? Panthers, leopards, lions, and tigers. They don't eat COW food. They are carnivores, and they eat protein. We are carnivores as well. You'll lean out quickly if you switch from COW food to protein.

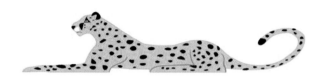

The key to ALL this **FAT** loss is a lifelong...
CHANGE OF EATING HABITS.

But are you really ready for that change? Addiction is addiction, whether you're talking about drugs, alcohol, or SUGAR. It all begins in your mind. Like sex, chocolate, and many drugs, SUGAR is believed by researchers to cause the brain to release dopamine in the pleasure centers of the brain, which then fuels the addiction.

According to the National Library of Medicine, daily bingeing on SUGAR repeatedly releases dopamine in the accumbens shell.

Simply spoken, SUGAR releases the "feel-good hormone" into your brain, fueling your desires for more SUGAR! It's a never-ending cycle. It's going to be completely up to you to re-train yourself to eat the foods that won't fuel your addiction and that won't make you **FAT**.

Your current eating habits are loaded with SUGAR. This is why the addiction has occurred in the first place, and this is why, at least up until now, being **FAT** has not been your fault. Now the question is, what are you going to do about it? Are you going to ignore the addiction like millions of others, or are you going to take action? Are you going to control your food intake with good choices? It's really easier than you might think. Most of the time, eating low-SUGAR is not about what you put *on* a plate as much as what you take *off* a plate. Use this book and labels to learn how to identify the SUGAR in the ingredients, and it will be easy for you to make those choices.

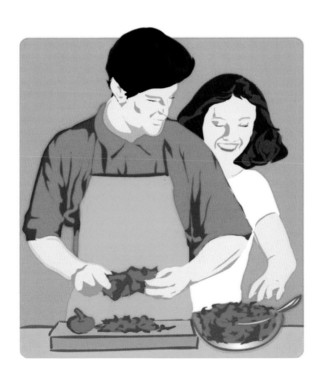

THE PSYCHOLOGICAL CONNECTION

Change is scary, even when it's for our own good. People like their *groove*; it fits like an old shoe. You not only have the issue of recognizing your SUGAR addiction to deal with, but you also have the other members of your household—who also have some level of SUGAR addiction—to deal with. They want to eat what *they* want to eat, not what you tell them to eat. Your problem is not their problem. To make matters worse, you'll have to take TOTAL charge of the foods that go into your mouth at home, at work, at dinner parties, and at restaurants. You'll need to be disciplined enough to stick to the good foods and have the strength to avoid the ones that have—and will continue to make you—**FAT**. Those foods will ALWAYS be at your fingertips wherever you go. In short, for you to succeed in your quest to become SKINNY, it needs to be important enough to you to make the appropriate changes in your eating habits.

Will it be difficult? All change comes with some level of difficulty; it depends on *your* personal commitment. For those of you who are determined to do something about your **FAT** problem once and for all, it will be easy, and you'll never be hungry. You simply have to make the changes required in your ingredient intake. Think of your personal battle with weight loss over the years. Us **FAT** people are willing to do just about anything to lose weight, except give up the foods we think we love.

I say "think" we love because you'll be amazed at how lousy white mashed potatoes, pasta, and white bread *really* taste once you remove them from your daily intake. But *wanting* to get SKINNY and *doing something* about getting SKINNY are totally separate issues. Millions of people *want* to be zillionaires, as long as it's a lottery win and they don't have to work for it. Millions of alcoholics *want* to quit drinking, but not bad enough to throw away the bottle. The amazing thing about getting rid of SUGAR is how simple the process is. The difficult part for most SUGAR addicts is actually doing it. Many people would rather do some of the things I have listed below. You may have tried one or several of the following methods yourself:

LOW-FAT DIETS

STARVING YOURSELF

TAKING DIET PILLS

AN ALL-LIQUID DIET

CONSIDERING LIPOSUCTION

KILLING YOURSELF IN THE GYM

CONSIDERING GASTRIC BYPASS

or worse

GIVING UP COMPLETELY!

In light of the above, spending a little time and effort on what you're actually eating that's *causing* your **FAT** problem doesn't seem so bad, now, does it? Think about it this way: if you were allergic to peanuts, and eating even the smallest amount could kill you, would you eat them? Of course not! And SUGAR *is* killing you as sure as peanuts kill some people. The only difference is that it's killing you *slowly*.

Eliminating SUGAR from your system will never be easier or better for you. You'll become thin and energetic, and you'll look and feel better, all without being hungry. You'll be able to dine out at most restaurants by giving instructions to the waitstaff. You'll be able to carry foods with you that will satisfy your body's needs without causing you to become **FAT**. You'll be able to enjoy many of your favorite recipes with some substitutions. This is your moment of truth. Moving forward from here can and will be your miracle, if you're ready for it.

What is your motivation to lose weight? Funny enough, mine was that one day I would no longer be a *special person*. I simply wanted to be a *normal person*, a person who could walk the beach in a Speedo bathing suit and not look ridiculous. Little did I know growing up that, as an adult, reaching the Speedo wish I had struggled with since I was eight or nine years old would be my motivator.

I have spoken to lots of people about motivation. Some are motivated because they want to live to play with their grandchildren. Some are motivated strictly by vanity or health. Others are motivated because they had given up and now see the possibility of finally getting SKINNY. Whatever your motivation, write it down on a Post-it note and stick it on your fridge. Find your goal-orientated self and charge forward.

My **FAT** friends thought I was crazy when I started eating low-SUGAR. I got all the negative comments. "Your heart's going to blow eating all that food!" "You're crazy! You can't eat all that food and lose weight!" Believe me, I enjoyed myself thoroughly as 50 pounds melted away like butter in a hot pan in just four months. My **FAT** melted so fast I actually had a friend ask me if I had contracted AIDS! I laughed, and we sat and talked about eating low-SUGAR/low-carb. The guy who was calling me crazy just a short four months earlier was now VERY curious about how I had lost all that **FAT**! He now wanted the secrets to losing his *ORB*. That's what he called his gut, his ORB. And his ORB was growing bigger every day. Five months later, he was 40 pounds lighter without exercise and while eating all the food he wanted. My friend dropped down to 175 pounds and ate ice cream all the way down! *Did I say ice cream?*

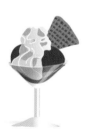

There is one more chemical issue to discuss with you. Remember what I said: you need to keep your **net** carbohydrate intake to under 20 grams per day to shed the **FAT**. There is a difference between carbohydrates and **net** carbohydrates. It's the word **NET** that we need to discuss. Some carbohydrates don't cause an insulin spike. Those carbs are SUGAR alcohols, artificial sweeteners, and fiber. When determining your carb counts in foods, you need to subtract SUGAR alcohols and fiber from the total carb count on labels to arrive at **net** carbs. This is important to you because it opens up many foods to you that otherwise would be avoided, including candy. Yes, I said candy. ALWAYS check the labels of everything you eat until the statistics are like second nature to you. Here's an example of a typical label and how you'll arrive at your net carb count:

NUTRITION FACTS

Serving size 1 bar (30 grams)

Calories	120
Calories from Fat	45
Total Fat	5g
Saturated Fat	3g
Trans fat	0g
Cholesterol	<5mg
Sodium	70mg
Total Carbohydrates	**15g**
Dietary Fiber	2g
Sugars	<1g
Sugar Alcohol	12g
Protein	6g

Total Carbohydrates   1 gram

This is a Slim Fast snack bar sweetened with the SUGAR alcohol Splenda. In this example, one bar is the serving size. Total carbs listed is 15 grams. Subtract 2 grams of fiber and 12 grams of SUGAR alcohol for a final net carb count of **1**. You could eat this bar and still have 19 grams of net carbs to play with for the day.

See how easy that was? **READ LABELS!** Here is a SUGAR-free Jell-O label—no carbs, no SUGAR!

NUTRITION FACTS

Serving size ¼ package (2.5 grams)

Calories	10
Total Fat	0g
Saturated Fat	0g
Trans Fat	0g
Sodium	55mg
Total Carbohydrates	**0g**
Sugars	0g
Protein	1g

Total Carbohydrates   0 grams

LET'S DISCUSS SUGAR ALCOHOLS AND ARTIFICIAL SWEETENERS

Okay, so you have a sweet tooth and find yourself in need of an occasional fix, what do you do? Obviously SUGAR is out of the question . . . but good news is on the horizon. You can have your sweets and still lose weight.

SUGAR alcohols and artificial sweeteners are what sweeten SUGAR-free products, including SUGAR-free candy, ice cream, and soda. They come in several forms, including stevia, maltitol, acesulfame potassium, sucralose (Splenda), sorbitol, saccharin, aspartame (Nutrasweet), mannitol, xylitol, lactitol, and isomalt.

There are a few things you should know about SUGAR alcohols and artificial sweeteners. First of all, they are reported not to have any significant effect on blood SUGAR. Some will, however, burn as fuel before **FAT** does. There are conflicting reports regarding their effects on different people. For example, some diabetics report a SUGAR *high* from some of these products, and some diabetic doctors require their patients to be wary of their use. I have been successful using these products as long as I keep them to a minimum. SUGAR-free products are your rewards and should be eaten as **occasional treats**, and not on a daily basis. It's also important to stay within the serving size. Most diet soda is sweetened with aspartame or Splenda. I prefer the Splenda-sweetened soda to the aspartame-sweetened soda. I've identified aspartame in my diet as a major cause of headaches, so I keep its use to a minimum.

Aspartame is by far the most controversial of all artificial sweeteners, so I'm going to spend a little extra time discussing it with you. Stories abound on the Web about its ill effects. As you read their stories, the authors will try to convince you that this artificial sweetener is as bad as ingesting radioactive material. I'm not a scientist, so I can only comment truthfully to you about my personal experience with the stuff. If you're experiencing headaches and using the little blue packets or drinking diet soda sweetened with aspartame, try eliminating them from your diet. You may be surprised when your headaches suddenly disappear.

Of course I wouldn't be satisfied advising you without some fairly exhaustive research on the subject. I went straight to the top and bypassed the doomsday articles written by *people*, many of whom are unqualified to write them in the first place. Instead I read study after study performed by scientists, clinical labs and medical professionals. What conclusion did I come to? The FDA, the manufacturer, and many clinical studies claim that aspartame is perfectly safe, while many reports, watchdog groups, and Web sites claim we are all being poisoned for the sake of corporate profits.

Who do you believe, the guys making money from the sales of product or the watchdog groups trying to save the world?

You decide. Below I've supplied you with the Web addresses for the manufacturer of aspartame, the FDA report on artificial sweeteners including aspartame, and the Web addresses for a couple of sites claiming aspartame is bad for you. I've also included the study performed by the National Cancer Institute. This will allow you to determine your personal position on aspartame. *My position* is simple: the stuff causes me headaches, so I don't use it. There are simply too many other products available sweetened with far less controversial sweeteners to choose from, so why take the chance?

SITES FOR ASPARTAME SAFETY

http://www.aboutaspartame.com/professional/index.asp

http://www.fda.gov/FDAC/features/1999/699_sugar.html

SITES CONDEMNING ASPARTAME

http://www.medicalnewstoday.com/articles/34040.php

http://www.holisticmed.com/aspartame/

NATIONAL CANCER INSTITUTE STUDY

http://www.cancer.gov/cancertopics/factsheet/risk/aspartame

Maltitol and sorbitol are major sweeteners in SUGAR-free candies, carb-free protein bars, and carb-free ice cream. The major side effect from these sweeteners is flatulence. Too much of a good thing will cause you to have gas (or worse), so take it easy and stay within the suggested serving size.

Stevia is my chosen sweetener; it's all natural, it has no carbs in its pure form and therefore doesn't need to be counted. Stevia can be purchased at most health food stores in several forms. Be careful to check the labels on the form you choose. I have found stevia in packets that have additional ingredients added to create more of a granular effect. It's the additional ingredients that can bring carbs into the product. In its raw form, it's more like baby powder. I sweeten my coffee, so I prefer the stevia tablets. I buy them on the Web at **www.sweetleaf.com**. They also sell the other forms of the product.

I recommend you limit your SUGAR-free sodas to no more than four per day, spread out through the day. Make water your main source of hydration. What I do is open a can of soda and top off my water glass with a splash of soda. One can of soda goes a long way using this method. You can eat a measured serving of Breyers CarbSmart ice cream or SUGAR-free candy no more than three times per week. I enjoy a serving of SUGAR-free Jell-O topped with Reddi-wip more than any of the other desserts. This dessert can be eaten every day.

If your weight loss plateaus for longer than two weeks, eliminate ALL SUGAR alcohol and artificially sweetened products from your intake. Once you start dropping weight again, slowly add back the *necessary* products and keep an eye on the scale. You may discover some sweeteners affect your weight and others don't.

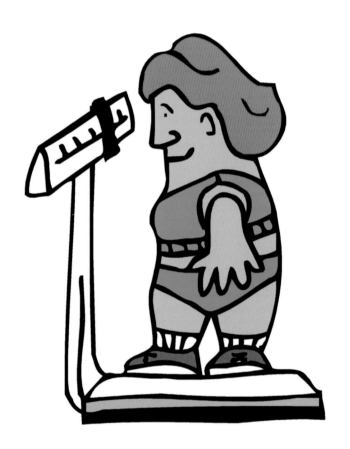

EATING YOURSELF SKINNY

By now you're probably asking yourself what you'll be able to eat that will be good for you and not feed into your SUGAR addiction. Let's start with two rules:

Eat MEATS and GREENS to grow THIN and LEAN

Eat SUGAR and CARBS to grow FAT and LARGE

Coming up in the next chapter of this book is your new ingredient list for your household shopping. Before you go to the store, I want you to analyze ALL of the food in your house. Read EVERY label on every bit of food you have in your cabinets and refrigerator. It's time to clean house of all the stuff that's making you **FAT**. Box up EVERYTHING that has a net carb count of over 4 grams per serving. Remember, net carbs are arrived at by looking at the total carb count on the label and subtracting the fiber and the SUGAR alcohols. The SUGAR that's listed on the label is factored into the total carb count and is *not subtracted*. ***Only the fiber and the SUGAR alcohols get subtracted from the total carb count to arrive at net carbs.***

Next, return what you can to your grocery store and give the non-returnable, sealed items to charity. Throw the rest away! If you're going to shut off the SUGAR pipeline, it begins at home. Everyone in your home will benefit from this eating plan—even the thin people living with you. You can save those thin people from becoming **FAT**, unless of course you want them to experience being a *special person* at Joubert's. ☺

Next, take this book to the store and restock your house with ALL low-SUGAR foods. It's time to eat yourself SKINNY! Some products will not be available at your grocery store and will need to be ordered in by phone or over the Web. Get used to it; as the low-carb FAD dies away, so will the low-carb products being carried in your local store. For us, shopping on the Web has become part of the norm. To make it easier for you, I have provided you with the ordering information. A word of caution: ***carefully read labels***. Something advertised as "SUGAR-free" may still be loaded with hidden SUGAR. The only measurement that's important to you is the NET CARBOHYDRATE COUNT.

SAMPLE LABEL

Total Carbohydrates	24g
Dietary Fiber	6g
Sugar	5g
Sugar Alcohols	10g
NET CARBS	8g

Carbs (24) – [Fiber (6) + SUGAR Alcohols (10)] = 8

WHEN SHOULD YOU EAT?

When you eat and how much you eat is determined by your activity level and your portion control. Whoever came up with the ritual of breakfast, lunch, and dinner based on the clock was an idiot. Your body requires energy to burn when you're burning energy. It doesn't require high doses of food if you're sedentary, any more than your car requires more gas when it's not running. Take the BEAR, for example. During hibernation, the bear slows down its metabolism and lives on body **FAT**. Are you hibernating or are you running all day long? Active people will need to eat more frequently than non-active people.

Before we discuss suggested eating times and quantities, let's discuss hunger. Do you know what the feeling of hunger is? Are you eating because it's your lunch break, or are you eating because you're hungry? Does your body tell you you're hungry and *then* you think of food, or do you think of food and *then* become hungry? For example, have you ever walked past a bakery and smelled *that bakery smell* and THEN said, "That smells wonderful. I'm hungry"? That's an example of food giving you false hunger. An example of true hunger is when your body interrupts you with signals and actually *tells you it's hungry. Note: a growling stomach may be a false signal of hunger brought on by years of scheduled feedings.* The best way to determine when you're truly hungry is to experience hunger in your own body and learn from the signals. For some people, stomach growls are enough. Others experience a feeling of low energy, others get cold, and others get grumpy.

The best thing to do is start off with a three-day test. (Yes, you need a paper and pencil.) Start your morning off with a small breakfast of two eggs, three strips of bacon or ham, and two pieces of GG Bran CrispBread with two tablespoons of the peanut butter mixture from page 108 in the ingredient section. For a beverage, drink whatever you want as long as it's SUGAR-free. Now write down the time you ate. Next, head into your day and see what happens. When you start to feel hunger, analyze it. Is it hunger or habit? Did you start thinking of food and that's what made you feel hungry, or were you interrupted by your body *telling you* you're hungry?

If your body has interrupted you from your work and told you you're hungry, then listen to it. If you started thinking about food and *then* became hungry, then you're experiencing a craving. Either way, write down the time on your paper and note whether it's true hunger or a craving. If it's a craving, drink a large glass of water or two and the craving will pass. If it's hunger, it will come back fairly quickly. If it's true hunger, have a small snack from any of the items on your ingredient list on page 97. It doesn't matter whether it's a handful of almonds, a couple of pieces of beef jerky, a hard-boiled egg, or items from the veggie tray. Now wait 15 to 20 minutes for the body to register the food and see how you feel. If you're satisfied the hunger has passed, make a note of what time you ate, what you ate, and the quantity of what you ate. If you're still hungry after 20 minutes, eat a little bit more and wait another 15 minutes, making notes along the way.

Once you've satisfied your hunger, it's time to wait for the body to signal you again. You may not hear from your body for another four or five hours, or you may hear from your body within two hours. It all depends on your activity level. Ignore the traditional breakfast, lunch, and dinner schedule for three full days.

The only scheduled meal I want you to eat during this experiment is breakfast, and I don't want you to eat *that* until you're hungry! It may be 10 a.m. before your body is asking for food. If you get an early start in the morning and usually don't eat breakfast until 10 a.m., that's okay. Hard-boiled eggs are the same as fried eggs, and you can carry them with you. Eat when you get your first *true* hunger. That will start your day with a timeline to work from. If you reach lunchtime and find you're not truly hungry, don't eat! Wait for the signals. It may be two in the afternoon before you feel hunger. That's when you'll eat another snack, and then wait for the signals again. Again, keep a log of your body's commands and responses.

After continuing with this experiment for three full days, you'll know when your feeding times are based on your log and the responses your body had to the food. Your goal during this three-day experiment is to put yourself in direct contact with your body's true feeding times versus cravings, and to identify the true quantity of food your body requires to satisfy those needs.

Once you have finished your experiment, look at the feeding schedule you experienced over three days. You should discover that you get urges to eat at about the same time each day. You'll also discover that it doesn't take much food to satisfy your needs during those times. Now you can custom-schedule *your* feedings to *your* feeding times, and maybe even rejoin the lunch and dinner crowd. To rejoin the lunch and dinner crowd, analyze your snack times and see how they coincide with the scheduled lunch and dinner breaks. For example, if you ate your breakfast at 8:30 a.m. and didn't get hungry again until 11 a.m. during your three-day experiment, you know that your body gets hungry an hour before the noon lunch break. You'll deal with this by eating a small amount at 11 a.m. Now, when lunchtime rolls around, you won't feel ravenous and you'll eat a smaller feeding at lunchtime. Three hours later your next feeding time may come up from your log. That's okay—have a small snack from the list to tide you over until dinner, and then eat a smaller dinner.

For Sherri and me, our eating schedule is as follows:

GG Bran CrispBread & peanut butter mixture with

coffee—7 a.m.
Breakfast or brunch—between 10 a.m. and 11 a.m.
Snacks—between 2 p.m. and 3 p.m.
Dinner—between 5 p.m. and 6 p.m.
Ice cream or Jell-O—8 p.m.

We eat five smaller meals per day instead of three big meals. Each of you will be different based on your experiment. Once you know your personal hunger schedule, you'll be prepared for it and will have food ready to eat on time. This will stop the ravenous search for something to eat when you're over-hungry and couldn't care less what goes into your mouth.

Don't let anyone make you feel that you're doing something wrong if you don't sit down at the food trough on someone else's schedule. This is *your* body, *your* schedule. There's nothing antisocial about it. You do what's right for you, not what's right for someone else. Just because dinner is on the table doesn't mean that you have to join in the feed. If you're not truly hungry, don't eat! Once you begin this practice you'll get to know your timelines so well that you'll never be hungry again. You'll eat when you first sense the feelings, satisfying your needs. And you'll never be ravenous.

During your experiment, you may also discover other reasons that you're eating. It's important to recognize the signs, because you may be *emotionally* eating. Pain seeks pleasure, and for SUGAR addicts, food *is* pleasure. If you find yourself seeking food because you're mad or upset, sad or stressed-out, then you're seeking pleasure from food to reverse the pain from the event. You are *emotionally* eating. This is simply a habit, and all habits can be broken if you recognize them. The trick is to replace the bad habit with a good habit. Find something besides food to bring you pleasure in times like these. Learn to eat for the right reasons. My personal demon is *nervous* eating. I call it "mindless" eating because I'm doing it without realizing it. If I have anxiety about something, I find myself strolling around the kitchen (and inevitably, to the fridge). For me, it's imperative to "bullet-proof" my kitchen and my fridge with SUGAR-free snacks.

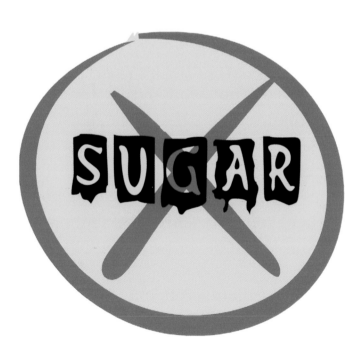

I'M STARVING!
TIME FOR A SNACK.

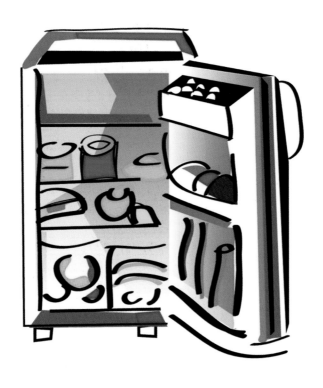

You've read a lot, I've written a lot. Let's share a snack together. I'll show you how easy it can be. Take me to your fridge!

Eating low-SUGAR is all about choices. Look for lunch meats like ham or sliced turkey. Grab the sliced cheese and the jar of pickles. Put all that stuff on the counter. Now lay out a piece of sandwich meat on a plate. On top of that, put a piece of cheese. Now lay a ¼ pickle slice on top of the cheese and roll the whole thing up like a sleeping bag. Congratulations, you're a chef! You just made a "meat, pickle, and cheese rollup." The only place SUGAR can be is if the meat is glazed with SUGAR or if there's SUGAR in the pickles. Check the labels. Buy SUGAR-free dill pickles, and deli meats without any SUGAR or honey glaze. Mix and match and include olives, if you wish. Keep rollups in the fridge ALL the time so you have something to grab when you're hungry.

Are you ready for another one?

Take out the eggs and hard-boil them. Once they're cooled and peeled, you can enjoy them whole with salt and pepper. Or you can make deviled eggs by cutting them in half lengthwise, taking out the yolk, mixing the yolks with some mayo (check the label), and stuffing the mixture back into the egg white. BINGO, deviled eggs! Keep these at your fingertips, too.

Got any hot dogs? Grab one and pop it in a microwave-safe bowl with a little water in the bottom. Cover and microwave for a couple of minutes.

Take out a head of lettuce and peel off a big leaf. Put in some mustard, put in your hot dog, roll it up, and eat it. Your catsup is probably full of SUGAR, so check the label. If you like catsup, buy SUGAR-free catsup. It's available at most stores.

While the lettuce and the lunchmeat and the boiled eggs are still out, let's make a nice big chef's salad for lunch. Put a mess of greens into a bowl, top it off with slivers of meats and cheeses and a hard-boiled egg. Check the dressings in the fridge. A lot of your favorites already in there are probably low-carb.

Do you have any shrimp in the freezer? Boil some up in Old Bay seasoning and leave them in the fridge to snack on. Mix some of that SUGAR-free catsup with some horseradish to make a SUGAR-free cocktail sauce. Let's check the veggie drawer. Pull out the broccoli, celery, cucumber, radishes, yellow squash, and the zucchini. Cut up a nice mix of this stuff and make yourself a low-SUGAR veggie tray. Use the low-SUGAR dressings in the fridge as a dip.

Let's check the freezer. See any boneless chicken breasts? Take a couple out and pan-fry them in some olive oil. Once cooled, slice them up, put some salt and pepper on them, and keep them in a bowl in the fridge. While we're in the freezer, let's check on steak. If you see a steak in the freezer, slice it up and then stick the meat strips on bamboo skewers. These are great grilled and left in the fridge. We love "meat on a stick!" If, by chance, you have any Walden Farms SUGAR-free BBQ sauce in the cabinet, brush some on during grilling.

We have lots of stuff out on the counter, so let's make one more thing together. Let's make kabobs! All you have to do is put chunks of chicken or steak on skewers along with chunks of yellow and green squash, a piece of onion, a couple of pieces of bell pepper, and on the grill they go.

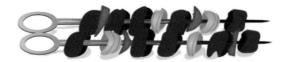

See how easy that was? Your fridge is now LOADED with healthy SUGAR-free and low-SUGAR treats. Get into the habit of making your own snack trays every day so you always have picking food. A mixture of these items can end up in your fridge at the office very easily.

When planning meals, plan on a main ingredient that can be used in different dishes for a couple of days. For example, let's say you plan a baked ham for Sunday dinner. Monday could be ham and eggs for breakfast, and *chicken cordon bleu* for dinner. *Chicken cordon bleu* is a chicken breast stuffed with ham and Swiss cheese, then baked. You'll find the recipe in the recipe section of this book. While you're making your *chicken cordon bleu*, prepare two or three extras. That way, you can slice them into pinwheels the next day and put them on a snack tray. Preparing food will become a habit for you. If you don't like to cook and prefer eating out, I have prepared a chapter further on in the book just for you.

INGREDIENT LIST

If you encounter problems with any product Web addresses, refer to our Web site for updates.

DINNERS and LUNCHES

Fresh MEATS, POULTRY, FISH

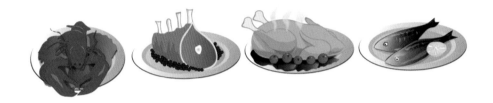

Buy any kind of meat, poultry, or fish you want, as long as it's lean, fresh, and not processed with store marinades or coatings. They are all *0 net carbs*. **Try to keep your serving size to 6 oz, but if you're still hungry after 15 minutes, EAT MORE.**

Carb-free doesn't mean calorie-free, and although this eating plan does not require you to count calories, portion sizes should be controlled to avoid gluttony. It takes the body longer to recognize the "full" feeling from protein, so try to eat a little slower and use the "15-minute rule" before refilling your plate with second helpings. Most people will feel full within 15 minutes with a 6-oz portion of protein.

Think of it. Steaks, chops, turkey, chicken, pork, roasts, salmon, grouper, shrimp, crab, tuna, crawfish, veal, lamb, and all the other wonderful non-processed fresh meats, poultry, and fish products contain ZERO SUGAR! Your dinner plate is starting off well, don't you think? Side the meat, poultry, or fish with a nice salad and any of the vegetables on the upcoming list for a complete, well-balanced, virtually SUGAR-free meal! Make wonderful chef's salads for lunches with GG Bran CrispBread as a side. Finish with a dessert of fresh strawberries, blackberries, or raspberries topped with Reddi-wip topping! Or, if you prefer, a ½-cup portion of Breyers CarbSmart ice cream or SUGAR-free Jell-O with Reddi-wip topping!

BREAKFASTS

BACON, SAUSAGE, AND HAM

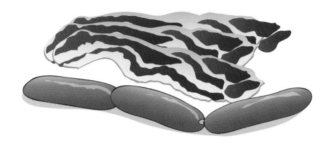

Most bacon, sausage, and ham are zero (or very low) in net carbs. **Check the labels** and beware of *SUGAR-cured* or *SUGAR-coated* products; they are loaded with carbs. I also still practice eating foods with the lowest possible **FAT** content to maintain healthy cholesterol levels. Buy leaner cuts and lower **FAT**-content products as long as there is no added SUGAR. Enjoy bacon and eggs for breakfast as often as you wish. Help control cholesterol by substituting whole eggs with Egg Beaters, and replace pork bacon with Louis Rich Turkey Bacon. Replace the toast with GG Bran CrispBread. Enjoy cheese omelets and soufflés. On the run, make BLTs and breakfast wraps made in La Tortilla Factory tortillas or wrapped in romaine leaves.

EGGS, EGG BEATERS, AND CHEESES

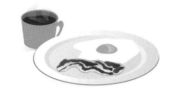

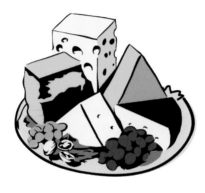

Buy any kind you want—they are all very low or *0 net carbs*, except for some **FAT**-free cheeses. Check the labels, and if they are under 2 net carbs per serving, they're okay. Discover the world of fine cheeses. You'll be amazed at the variety and selection of cheeses from around the world to explore, all of them SUGAR-free and loaded with calcium. To control cholesterol, limit whole eggs by using egg substitutes, such as Egg Beaters, and watch your portion sizes with full-**FAT** cheeses. Info on Egg Beaters can be found at **www.eggbeaters.com**.

BEVERAGES

WATER   *0 net carbs*
DIET SODA   *0 net carbs, limit to 4 per day*

Stick with brands of diet soda sweetened with Splenda or stevia; stay away from aspartame. Diet Rite made by RC Cola has 4 flavors: cola, white grape, black cherry, and orange. Coke and Pepsi also have certain sodas with Splenda.

Herbal teas   *0 net carbs*
Black coffee   *1 net carb*
Wyler's Light   *1 net carb*
Crystal Light   *1 net carb*

Lighten coffee with half & half (1 tbsp)   *.5 net carbs*
or heavy whipping cream   *0 net carbs*
Sweeten with stevia tabs   *0 net carbs*

BREADS

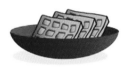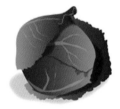

You'll need no other kind of bread besides GG Bran CrispBread and La Tortilla Factory tortillas, and nice crisp romaine lettuce leaves. There are several *crisp breads* on the market, many of them loaded with SUGAR, so I want you to buy the one I recommend. Order a case over the Web and use it for peanut butter crackers, cheese and crackers, cream cheese and jelly, peanut butter and jelly (Frugeli brand jelly), or simply with butter or olive oil alongside a meal or salad. They are 100% bran, so they give you a good dose of fiber.

La Tortilla Factory tortillas are wonderful and come in three flavors. They are probably available from your local health food store or better grocery store, but if not, I've supplied the Web address. They make terrific wraps for sandwiches. They also make great enchiladas and fajitas. We also use nice big fresh romaine lettuce leaves as a wrapper. We fill them with ham, turkey, salami, and cheeses for fulfilling sandwiches that are totally carb-free. They also make for a great hamburger or hot dog bun replacement.

GG Bran CrispBread *2 net carbs*
www.brancrispbread.com

La Tortilla Factory Tortilla *3 net carbs*
www.latortillafactory.com

DESSERTS and JELLY

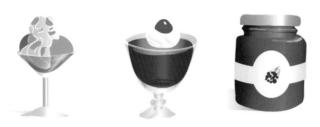

YES, desserts! Eat in moderation. I know you have a sweet tooth, so I've provided you with some prepackaged products sweetened with SUGAR alcohols or artificial sweeteners. Remember what I said about SUGAR alcohols: they are self-policing. Eat too many and they will cause a laxative affect. Stay within the portion size once or twice a day and you'll be fine.

Tastykake Sugar Free Sensables
Chocolate Chip Cake   *4 net carbs*
Chocolate Cake   *2 net carbs*
www.tastykake.com
Also available at Publix stores & Walmart.

Miss Meringue Sugar-free Meringue Cookies
Chocolate and vanilla all *0 net carbs*
www.missmeringue.com/Sugar-Free/c/Miss
Meringue@SugarFree

Fifty-50 Fruit Spreads
Available in 3 flavors: grape, raspberry, strawberry, orange, blackberry, and apricot
1 net carb or less per serving
www.fifty50foods.com/spreads.html

ICE CREAM, JELL-O, and WHIPPED CREAM

Available at most grocery stores

Breyers CarbSmart (½ cup) *4 net carbs*
Vanilla, butter pecan, chocolate, and rocky road.
You'll find these products on their Web site under the Breyers tab/packaged ice cream.
www.icecreamusa.com

Blue Bunny No Sugar Added (½ cup) *3 net carbs*
Peanut butter fudge, chocolate almond fudge. You'll find these flavors on their Web site under Lighter Options/ No Sugar Added, Reduced Fat Products.
www.bluebunny.com

Jell-O brand SUGAR-free gelatin *0 net carbs*
www.kraftfoods.com/jello/

Reddi-wip canned real whipped cream topping *<1 net carb*
www.reddi-wip.com

CANDY and COOKIES

Russell Stover SUGAR-free candy is wonderful. So are the **Hershey's** brand candies. Walmart stores carry both brands.
www.russellstover.com
www.hersheys.com

Miss Meringue Sugar-free Meringues *0 net carbs*
Chocolate and vanilla
www.missmeringue.com/Sugar-Free/c/Miss
Meringue@SugarFree
Beanit Butter Walnut Cookies *0 net carbs*
Recipe in recipe section on page 262.

FRUIT

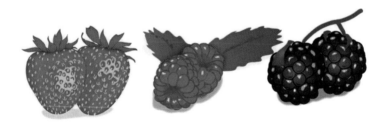

Fresh or frozen berries and avocados are the only fruits you're allowed until you've lost ALL the **FAT** you want. At that point, you can slowly add some of the other lower SUGAR fruits into your diet, such as apples, watermelon, cantaloupe, honeydew, apricots, and peaches. The following counts are for ½ cup servings unless otherwise noted:

Strawberries   **3.5 net carbs**
Blackberries   **5.5 net carbs**
Raspberries   **3 net carbs**
Avocado (small)   **2 net carbs**

MUFFIN and PANCAKE MIXES

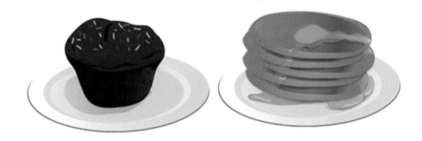

Top with cream cheese for a delicious treat.

Dixie Carb Counters
Banana nut muffin (1) *4 net carbs*
Carrot muffin (1) *1 net carb*
Cranberry orange muffin (1) *4 net carbs*
www.dixiediner.com

New Hope Mills Low Carb Sugar-Free Pancake & Waffle Mix
(4 pancakes) *3 net carbs*
www.carbsmart.com

Log Cabin Sugar-Free Syrup
(¼ cup) *0 net carbs*
Available at most grocery stores

NUTS, CHIPS, and PEANUT BUTTER

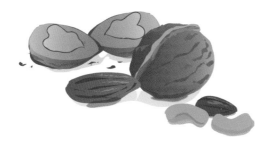

Dry Roasted Edamame (¼ cup) *2 net carbs*
www.seapointfarms.com

Almonds (30) *2.5 net carbs*

Walnuts (¼ cup) *1 net carb*

EatSmart Soy Crisps (10) *3 net carbs*
www.eatsmartsnacks.com

Pork Skins, fried, unsweetened *0 net carbs*

Peanut Butter, soy *0 net carbs*

Carb Not Beanit Butter *0 net carbs*
www.dixiediner.com
Order number (1-800-233-3668)

Smucker's Chunky Natural Peanut Butter
(2 tablespoons) *4 net carbs*

Doug's Crunchy Peanut Butter Mix—one 15 oz jar of Carb Not Beanit Butter mixed with one 16 oz jar of Smucker's Chunky Natural Peanut Butter and ½ cup chopped Dry Roasted Edamame (2 tbsp) *2 net carbs*

PROTEIN BARS

You have to be careful with protein bars. Many are loaded with SUGAR. I recommend the following:

Optimum Nutrition Complete Protein Diet Bars (1 bar) *1 net carb*
www.optimumnutrition.com

SAUCES and SALAD DRESSING

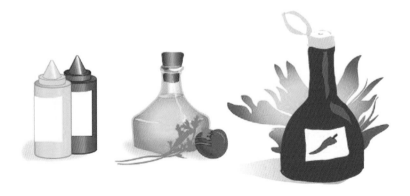

Walden Farms BBQ Sauces *0 net carbs*
www.waldenfarms.com

Winn-Dixie Pasta Sauce (¼ cup) *2 net carbs*

Emeril's Roasted Red Pepper Pasta Sauce (¼ cup) *2.5 net carbs*
www.everythingemeril.com

Heinz Classic Chicken Gravy (¼ cup) *3 net carbs*

Tabasco Hot Sauce *0 net carbs*

Cholula Hot Sauce *0 net carbs*

Bertolli Alfredo Sauce (¼ cup) *3 net carbs*
www.bertolli.com

Many brand-name salad dressings are already low in SUGAR. Check the labels on your favorites. Here are some examples:

Kraft Seven Seas (2 tbsp) *2 net carbs*

Kraft Classic Caesar (2 tbsp) *<1 net carb*

Wish-Bone Carb-Options Blue Cheese (2 tbsp) *0 net carbs*

Athenos Greek with Feta Cheese (2 tbsp) *2 net carbs*

Sour cream (2 tbsp) *1 net carb*

PASTA

Tofu Shirataki Pasta (1 cup) *2 net carbs*
www.house-foods.com

VEGETABLES

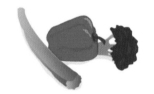

Look at the incredible amount of variety in your veggie list, all of it low in SUGAR! Get creative with your veggies. Make meat or seafood stir-fries, enjoy delectable chef's salads with eggs, cheeses, and meats. Enjoy steamed cauliflower run through your food processor as a mashed potato replacement. Enjoy spaghetti squash, julienned zucchini, or Tofu Shirataki Pasta as a replacement for pasta. Or simply enjoy veggie trays with ranch dressing as an anytime snack.

Counts are for ½ cup servings unless otherwise noted:

Artichoke hearts	*2 net carbs*
Asparagus, fresh (5 spears)	*2 net carbs*
Beans, green, fresh	*3 net carbs*
Bean sprouts	*2 net carbs*
Bok choy	*.2 net carbs*
Broccoli, fresh	*2 net carbs*

Cabbage, all kinds	*1.5 net carbs*
Cauliflower	*1.5 net carbs*
Celery (2 stalks)	*1.5 net carbs*
Chard, Swiss	*1.5 net carbs*
Chayote squash	*2 net carbs*
Collard greens	*2 net carbs*
Cucumber	*1 net carb*
Eggplant	*2 net carbs*
Fennel	*2 net carbs*
Garlic (1 clove)	*1 net carb*
Jicama	*2.5 net carbs*
Lettuce	*.5 net carbs*
Mushrooms	*2 net carbs*
Okra	*3 net carbs*
Onions	*5 net carbs*
Peppers, red or green bell	*3 net carbs*
Pumpkin meat	*4 net carbs*
Radicchio	*1 net carb*
Radishes	*1 net carb*
Scallions	*2.5 net carbs*
Snow peas	*3.4 net carbs*
Spinach, fresh	*.3 net carbs*
Spinach, frozen	*2 net carbs*
Squash, spaghetti	*4 net carbs*
Squash, yellow	*1.5 net carbs*
Squash, zucchini	*1.5 net carbs*
Tofu	*2.5 net carbs*
Tomato (1 small)	*3 net carbs*
Turnip	*2.5 net carbs*
Turnip greens	*1 net carb*
Watercress	*0 net carbs*

THE FOOD

When my book publisher came to me and asked me for 100 new recipes for this updated and revised edition of *FAT TO SKINNY: Fast and Easy!*, I was thrilled! Great low-sugar food is the foundation of the FAT TO SKINNY lifestyle, and eating great while losing weight is a blast.

As you can see from your ingredient list on page 97, there is no lack of food variety. What *is* missing are pre-made, processed foods and SUGAR. With the grocery list, you can mix and match tons of recipes using good, fresh food low in SUGAR and high in vitamins and minerals. Yes, it requires you to cook and to prepare food, but so what? Isn't it time you took control of what goes into your body? For years the food you've been eating has made and kept you **FAT** and unhealthy. Learning how to prepare your food and sticking to the FAT TO SKINNY lifestyle will make and keep you thin and healthy.

I've made it easy by providing you with lots of personal recipes that have been cooked in my own kitchen and enjoyed by my family and friends. Using these recipes for the whole family and for dinner parties will thrill and surprise even those without a weight problem. The foods we use are delicious, and the menu is diverse. There's no reason to cook different meals for others in your household. *You* buy the groceries and, trust me, they'll eat what you serve them. This way you'll keep yourself away from the temptation of foods that you know are unhealthy for you. You don't have to be a master chef, either; all you need to do is buy the ingredients and follow the step-by-step instructions. YES, it's that easy!

I've organized the cookbook section into the following categories:

1—Snack Trays, Appetizers, and Niblits
2—Breakfast
3—Lunch
4—Dinner
5—Dessert

As you browse through the recipes trying to decide where to begin, I suggest you start with a dinner. Pick a recipe that will give you leftovers for snack trays and lunches. This way, you provide yourself with the components for a few meals. Cooking doesn't have to be a chore; in fact, cooking should be and will be fun with a bit of advance planning.

Read the recipe first, then look in your freezer and pantry to see what you have on hand. Next, write out a grocery list for your trip to the store. Make sure you have the proper cooking utensils and pans for your chosen recipe. If the recipe calls for advance preparation, make certain you have enough time to pull it off. Finally, check the carb count on the recipe to see if it fits into your daily menu total. Remember the rule: stay 20 net carbs or under for the entire day's worth of food and beverages in order to lose weight. I have broken down the carb counts for the individual ingredients in each recipe so you can omit or reduce ingredients and make adjustments if you wish.

The last thing I want you to experience in the kitchen is frustration. Following the simple rules outlined above will help make your cooking an enjoyable experience.

So if you're ready to start, take me into the kitchen and let's get cooking!

I did mention I was a chef didn't I? Yes, I'm quite sure I did.

It's time to

EAT GREAT AND LOSE WEIGHT!

For FREE reader support visit **www.FATtoSKINNY.net**

TIP—My name is Tipster. Look for me throughout the book for cooking tips. Look for my video camera icon below for selected Web-supported recipes.

Video-supported recipe! Go to this Web site to watch me make it for you.
www.FATtoSKINNY.com/recipes.htm

The Basics

When I was just a lad growing up, I loved two chefs: Graham Kerr, also known as the Galloping Gourmet, and Julia Child. When Julia died in August 2004 I was heartbroken, for she represented the simplicity of the kitchen for me. Graham represented the fun aspect of the kitchen. It was a very cool mix that motivated me, even at the tender age of 12, to cook in my mom's kitchen. Well, that and the fact that I *loved* to eat and Mom, being a very busy businesswoman, didn't always have the time to cook. SpaghettiOs and canned ravioli just didn't do it for me, so it was time to take control! Julia and Graham showed me the way to great food. All I needed to do was write the ingredients on Mom's shopping list and bingo, they would magically arrive.

A few years ago I visited the Smithsonian National Museum of American History in Washington, DC, and discovered to my delight that Julia had donated her kitchen to the museum. Now, I'm not just talking about her pots and pans, I'm talking about her *entire kitchen*, including the walls, appliances, and everything else in it! It was a great experience for a guy who used to skip school and play sick just so I could stay home and watch my favorite chefs on TV. (Recording the shows wasn't an option back then; the technology didn't exist.) Visiting Julia's kitchen was a wonderful experience and I would like to share it with you. You don't even have to leave home and travel to Washington, DC, to see it, all you need to do is visit this link: **americanhistory.si.edu/juliachild/**.

What you'll find in Julia's kitchen is pure simplicity—nothing fancy. Expensive pots and pans, fancy tools, and high-end appliances don't make the chef. All you need is a heat source, a few basic pots and pans, a few basic tools, and the desire to eat great food. These are the elements of a great cook.

Your kitchen should be simple and easy to maneuver around. The tools you need should be easy to grasp and the kitchen should flow. *FUN* should be your goal in your kitchen. Graham cracked me up all the time with his whimsical jokes and the easy way about him. He took all the intimidation away from the task at hand . . . he made all things *EASY* in the kitchen.

Over the years I've developed *EASY* recipes that flow as easily as my kitchen. From last night's dinner to making use of the leftovers in tomorrow's breakfast, from doubling a recipe for an entrée to a snack tray, it all flows. In the following pages I've included tips to teach you this flow. Make it easy on yourself and the fun part will be automatic.

Savory was Julia's trademark. Being a French chef, Julia used butter and cream, cheeses, and spices to magically whip up recipes that delighted and amazed me.

Healthy comes in when a recipe works in concert with your body to feed your body's needs in a balanced fashion. Discovering *healthy* came to me much later in life, not until my forties in fact. My focus in the kitchen simply revolved around taste and appetite satisfaction. I've noticed the same thing seems to be true even in today's televised kitchens. Ever notice how your favorite TV chefs are getting *fatter* and FATTER and **FAT**? I won't mention any names . . . but you know who I'm talking about.

Let's take a few minutes and concentrate on *healthy*— after all, that's why you bought this book.

The recipes in this book are all designed to incorporate all four elements, while coaxing your body to shed those unwanted pounds. As explained earlier, sugar is your enemy. It's sugar and the foods that metabolize into sugar that have been and still are making you fat. My recipes carve the sugar away, forcing your body to burn your fat. Beware of the simple mistakes that will sabotage you in your quest to lose weight. It's important to stick to some simple rules.

The Rules

#1—STICK TO THE RECIPES.

Avoid substituting or adding non-listed ingredients. It's amazing, for example, how much sugar can be found in simple condiments like ketchup or certain salad dressings like raspberry vinaigrette or French.

#2—STAY UNDER 5 TEASPOONS OF SUGAR PER DAY.

To eat great and lose weight, stay under 5 teaspoons of sugar per day, which represents 20 carbs. Stay under that threshold and your body will be forced to use your stored fat as fuel.

#3—DON'T EAT WHILE YOU COOK!

Yes, I know that's tough, so I'll provide you the answer . . . chew sugar-free gum while you're cooking. To taste a recipe simply remove the gum, drink some water, and take a *small* taste. You can even spit it out if you wish.

#4—LEARN YOUR FOOD.

Review pages 78–79, where I taught you how to read nutritional labels, to make it easy for you to spot the hidden sugar in your ingredients.

Now I want you to take a moment and look at the food you have in your house. Let's go to the pantry first. See that box of cereal or that bag of flour or maybe that loaf of "healthy" wheat bread? Check out the label . . . go ahead, it won't bite—after today it will never hurt you again.

Are you shocked? All this time you thought you were eating healthy. Did you ever think for one second you were pouring all that sugar into your body?

Now, grab the trash can and throw it all away! Take the unopened products back to the store or donate them to the food bank. For you, it's all poison.

Making the decision to remove all the products from your home that are making you **FAT** is the first step to changing your lifestyle and dropping that weight.

But what about your sweet tooth? Not to worry, just wait until you taste my double-chocolate macadamia nut fudge, my peanut butter fudge ice cream cake, or blackberry sorbet covered in whipped cream!

Remember that first ingredient in a great recipe, *fun*?

Is it truly possible that losing weight can be FUN?
YOU BET!
Let's start the fun with snack trays, appetizers, and niblits.

SNACK TRAYS, APPETIZERS, AND NIBLITS

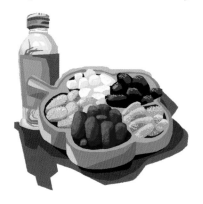

Snack trays are wonderful; they offer you bulletproof instant gratification. How many times have you opened the fridge door, stared in, and wondered what to eat? For most people, the next step is closing the fridge, opening the pantry, and grabbing the chips or cookies. Preparing snack trays on a continual rotating basis gives you an answer to the snatch-and-grab syndrome that is so typical among all of us who are carrying extra weight. The difference is, *now* when you snatch and grab, you'll be filling up with *fun, easy, healthy* foods that will promote weight loss, not weight gain. You will always have a variety of choices because you'll spin them out of the previous night's entrée on a continual basis.

For the times when you don't want to cook and instead choose the eat-out options, you can still have snack trays. Most supermarkets and delis have, or can prepare, any kind of tray you want. Veggie trays, meat trays, cheese trays, and chicken-wing trays are all very common.

Snack trays are *fun*! Here are some of my favorites.

Sweet-and-Sour Pork on a Stick

You will need about 25 12-inch bamboo skewers for the pork. I prefer black-berry or blueberry sugar-free pancake syrup for the kabobs.

Ingredients
½ cup fruit-flavored sugar-free pancake syrup
½ cup soy sauce (8 net carbs)
1 tablespoon Cajun Land Cajun Seasoning
1 tablespoon balsamic vinegar (2.5 net carbs)
2–3 packets stevia
2 pounds pork loin
2 small onions (10 net carbs)
2 medium bell peppers (6 net carbs)
1 cup shredded purple cabbage (3 net carbs)
¼ cup ranch dressing (2 net carbs)

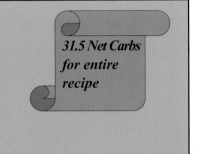

31.5 Net Carbs for entire recipe

1. Combine the following ingredients for the marinade: fruit-flavored pan-cake syrup, soy sauce, Cajun seasoning, stevia, and balsamic vinegar. Adjust for heat or sweet by adding additional Cajun seasoning or stevia to taste. If you want a little more sour, add additional vinegar, 1 teaspoon at a time.

2. Cut the pork loin into 1-inch-thick chops, then cut those chops into 1-inch-wide strips. You should now be looking at strips approximately 1 inch by 1 inch by 4 inches long. Place the strips in the marinade, making sure to cover all the surfaces, cover, and let stand in the refrigerator for 1 to 2 hours.

3. Count your strips and place an equal number of bamboo skewers in water. Keep them there until you remove the meat from the marinade.

4. Cut the onions and bell peppers into segments like an orange and set aside.

5. Prepare a serving platter by shredding the cabbage to cover the bottom of the dish.

6. Once the pork is done marinating, skewer the meat and vegetables on the prepared skewers, setting aside any leftover marinade for basting.

7. Heat up the grill and cook the kabobs to your desired doneness (see pork grilling chart on page 306), basting them once halfway through the cooking process. Since raw meat soaked in the marinade, make sure the marinade itself cooks for a bit. I prefer my pork medium rare; cooking it well done will dry it out.

8. Present the kabobs on the shredded cabbage with ranch dressing on the side. Mix the ranch dressing into the cabbage and use it as a dip for the onions and peppers.

TIP—The meat for these kabobs freezes very well raw, offering you a quick, easy snack tray. Simply wrap any extra kabobs tightly in plastic wrap, making sure to seal the ends, and then freeze. When you're ready to cook them, add the veggies.

Peppered Steak on a Stick

I use London broil for this recipe. It's lean, uniform in shape, contains no gristle, and cooks quickly. However, if the meat is cut wrong, it will be very tough. Look at the steak and identify which direction the grain is going. You will want to slice the steak against the grain. If you've sliced it correctly, you should be able to pull the slice apart with very little effort. If you've sliced the steak with the grain, it will be very hard to pull apart. You will need about 25 12-inch bamboo skewers for the kabobs.

Ingredients
1 pound London broil
Black pepper
Nonstick cooking spray
2 small ripe tomatoes, sliced (6 net carbs)
2–3 fresh parsley sprigs, for garnish

6 Net Carbs for entire recipe

1. Soak the bamboo skewers in water while preparing the kabobs.

2. Cut the steak into strips approximately 1 inch by 1 inch by 4 inches long. Count the strips and make sure you have enough skewers soaking.

3. Slip the skewers through the strips of meat as if you were sewing the meat with the skewer. Lay the skewered steak on a platter and coarsely grind pepper on each side to your liking (I like heavily peppering).

4. Heat up the grill, and clean the grate with a brush to avoid sticking. Lightly spray nonstick cooking spray on the skewered sticks of beef, then lay the skewers flat on the hot grill surface. Cook quickly, following the beef grilling chart on page 300.

5. Present the kabobs on a serving platter with the tomato and parsley.

TIP—The meat for these kabobs freezes very well raw, offering you a quick, easy snack tray. Simply wrap any extra kabobs tightly in plastic wrap, making sure to seal the ends, and then freeze. You can cut out all the carbs by eliminating the tomato, making this a 0-carb snack tray.

Video-supported recipe! Go to this Web site and watch the Beef Jerky recipe to learn how to cut London broil: **www.FATtoSKINNY.com/ recipes.htm.**

Chipotle Pepper Drums with Blue Cheese Dip

McCormick Grill Mates Chipotle Pepper Marinade is available in the spice section at most supermarkets.

Ingredients
8 chicken drumsticks
½ cup Kraft blue cheese dressing (4 net carbs)
1 package McCormick Grill Mates Chipotle

6 Net Carbs for entire recipe

1. Heat up the grill.

2. Strip the skin off the chicken drumsticks and place them in a mixing bowl. Add the McCormick Grill Mates Chipotle Pepper Marinade (available in the spice section at most supermarkets) and toss to coat the drumsticks well.

3. Place the drumsticks on the grill surface and cook through (see poultry grilling chart on page 312).

4. Serve with blue cheese salad dressing as a dip.

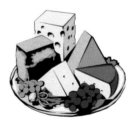 **TIP**—Cook extra drumsticks and freeze them in freezer bags for a quick snack or lunch. Most of the carbs in this recipe are from the dip.

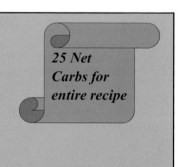

Antipasto Tray

Ingredients
Several wedges of different cheeses
1 red bell pepper (3 net carbs)
½ cup mixed olives (2 net carbs)
½ cup hot and mild peppers (2 net carbs)
½ cup raspberries (4 net carbs)
½ cup blackberries (4 net carbs)
½ cup strawberries (2 net carbs)
4 pieces GG Bran Crispbread, broken in half (8 net carbs)

25 Net Carbs for entire recipe

1. Lay out wedges of your favorite cheeses on an attractive tray.

2. Cut the bell pepper in half to use as two bowls. Fill the interior with your favorite olive and pepper mixes.

3. Decorate with the berries and serve with GG Bran Crispbread.

Chicken Pinwheels

Ingredients
2 slices ham
2 slices Swiss cheese
2 boneless, skinless chicken breasts
Salt and pepper

0 Net Carbs for entire recipe

1. Preheat the oven to 375 degrees.

2. Lay out a thin slice of ham. Place a slice of Swiss cheese on top of the ham and roll it up. Repeat with the remaining ham and cheese. Using a sharp knife, cut a pocket inside each chicken breast. Stuff the rolled ham and cheese into the pockets and close with wooden toothpicks. Season well with salt and pepper to taste and bake for 35 minutes.

3. Let the chicken cool completely in the fridge. Once cooled, slice each breast into ½-inch-thick pinwheels using a sharp knife. Arrange the pinwheels on a tray and bring them to room temperature before serving.

TIP—Slice pinwheels from extra chicken cordon bleu (see page 199) you made and refrigerated the evening before.

Chicken Wings, Hot and Spicy or BBQ

Buy the wings in the freezer section. They usually come in a 2½- or 5-pound bag. Be sure to get the uncoated kind. Many grocery stores now sell Walden Farms zero-carb products. Check out this link to purchase your BBQ sauce online or to find a retailer near you: **www.waldenfarms.com**.

Ingredients

2½ pounds frozen chicken wings

Salt

Cayenne pepper or Walden Farms BBQ Sauce

½ cup blue cheese dressing (4 net carbs)

4 large celery stalks, cut into sticks (3 net carbs)

1 tablespoon olive oil (to grease your cookie sheet)

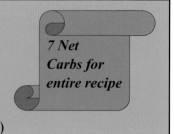

7 Net Carbs for entire recipe

1. Preheat the oven to 400 degrees.

2. Season the wings with salt and cayenne (be careful, it's HOT) or coat them with Walden Farms BBQ Sauce to your liking. Place the wings on a greased cookie sheet.

3. Bake the wings in the preheated oven. Turn once when golden brown and continue cooking until brown on top.

4. Serve with blue cheese dressing and celery sticks.

Prosciutto, Provolone, and Red Pepper Rollups

Buy thinly sliced prosciutto (salt-cured Italian ham) and provolone cheese from your local deli for this quick snack tray.

Ingredients

½ pound prosciutto, sliced

½ pound provolone cheese, sliced

1 red bell pepper, julienned (3 net carbs)

1 tablespoon extra-virgin olive oil

Cracked black pepper

2 teaspoons grated Romano cheese

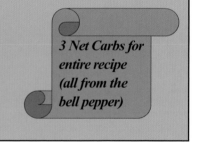

3 Net Carbs for entire recipe (all from the bell pepper)

1. Lay out a slice of ham, place a slice of cheese on top, then place a slice of bell pepper inside and roll up.

2. When you have made as many as you like, sprinkle each one with extra-virgin olive oil and a few grinds of pepper, and top with a sprinkling of Romano cheese. Let the rollups rest at room temperature for 20 minutes before serving.

Veggie Tray

You can use this list or any mix of veggies from the approved list (see page 110).

Ingredients
½ cup each of the following:
  Broccoli florets (2 net carbs)
  Cauliflower florets (1.5 net carbs)
  Celery (1.5 net carbs)
  Red bell pepper (3 net carbs)
  Green beans (3 net carbs)
  Zucchini (1.5 net carbs)
Salt
½ cup Hidden Valley Ranch dressing (4 net carbs)

16.5 Net Carbs for entire recipe

1. Cut up all the veggies into finger-food sizes.

2. Blanch the broccoli and cauliflower in boiling salted water for 60 seconds. Scoop out and immediately submerse the florets in ice water to stop the cooking process. Drain and pat the florets dry before arranging on a serving platter with the other veggies.

3. Serve with Hidden Valley Ranch salad dressing as a dip.

TIP—When you're chopping veggies, cut plenty extra and store them in a plastic bag in the fridge for quick, easy use.

Asparagus Snaps with Red Pepper and Sweet Lemon Dip

Serve this wonderful plate as a side dish with dinner or brunch or simply as a snack tray. Be sure to buy thin asparagus spears and a nice, crisp red bell pepper.

Ingredients

15 asparagus spears (6 net carbs)
4 tablespoons butter
Sea salt and pepper
1 medium red bell pepper (3 net carbs)
Juice of 1 lemon or 2 tablespoons bottled lemon
   juice (2.5 net carbs)
1–2 packets stevia

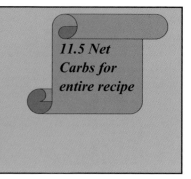

11.5 Net Carbs for entire recipe

1. Bring some salted water to a boil in a large saucepan on the stove. Cut 1 inch off the bottom of the asparagus spears to remove the tough, fibrous part. Drop the asparagus into the boiling water and cook for 2 minutes. Strain and leave in the sink.

2. Using the same pot, melt 1 tablespoon of the butter, then place the spears back into the pot and gently roll to coat with butter.

3. Transfer the asparagus to a serving plate and top with a tablespoon of butter and several grinds of salt and pepper. Cut the bell pepper into julienne strips and arrange them in an attractive design on top of the asparagus.

4. For the sweet lemon butter: Melt the remaining 2 tablespoons of butter and squeeze in the lemon juice. Add a packet of stevia and mix well. If you would like a sweeter taste, add another packet of stevia.

5. Serve the asparagus at room temperature with the dip.

Celery with Cream Cheese and Chopped Green Olives

Ingredients

¼ cup pitted, chopped green olives (2.5 net carbs)
½ cup cream cheese (3.5 net carbs)
4 large celery stalks (3 net carbs)
Freshly ground black pepper

9 Net Carbs for entire recipe

1. Mix the olives with the cream cheese.

2. Stuff the celery with the cream cheese mixture and grind a little pepper on top.

3. Cut the celery into bite-size pieces and keep refrigerated until ready to serve.

Cheese and Crackers

Ingredients
Cheddar cheese
Smoked Gouda cheese
Pepper jack cheese
Havarti cheese
2 strips bacon
2 scallions (.5 net carbs)
½ cup cream cheese (3.5 net carbs)
6 pieces GG Bran Crispbread (12 net carbs)

16 Net Carbs for entire recipe

1. Slice a variety of cheeses, such as cheddar, smoked Gouda, pepper jack, and Havarti, and arrange on a serving tray.

2. Pan-fry the bacon until crisp. Finely chop the bacon and the scallions and mix well with the cream cheese. Spoon the spread into a serving bowl and place the bowl in the middle of the serving tray.

3. Serve with GG Bran Crispbread.

Genoa Salami Rolls with Farmer Cheese and Roasted Garlic Spread

Ingredients
1 head garlic (1 net carb per large clove)
1 tablespoon olive oil
8 ounces farmer cheese

8 Net Carbs for entire recipe

2 tablespoons mayonnaise
¼ pound Genoa salami, sliced
½ cup pitted black olives (2 net carbs)

1. Preheat the oven to 350 degrees.

2. Cut the top quarter-inch off the head of garlic, place in an oven-safe dish, and drizzle the olive oil over the garlic. Bake the garlic for 20 to 25 minutes, or until soft when squeezed.

3. Crumble the farmer cheese into a mixing bowl and stir in the mayonnaise.

4. When the garlic cools, squeeze all the cloves into the cheese and mayonnaise mixture and mix well.

5. Place a teaspoon of filling into each piece of salami and roll it up. Stab a black olive with a toothpick and stick it into each roll.

6. Arrange the rolls on a serving tray and serve.

Caprese Salad—Mozzarella, Tomato, and Basil Plate

Buy fresh, vine-ripened tomatoes and fall in love with Italy all over again! The tomatoes for this dish should not be too wet or seedy; beefsteaks or even Italian plum do well.

Ingredients
1–2 tablespoons extra-virgin olive oil
2 small ripe tomatoes (6 net carbs)
Salt and cracked black pepper
8 ounces fresh mozzarella cheese
3–4 fresh basil leaves, chopped

6 Net Carbs for entire recipe

1. Pour some olive oil on a serving dish. Slice the tomatoes into nice thick slices and place on the oil. Flip the tomatoes over and gently salt and pepper. (You'll be using salt and pepper again, so go easy this time.)

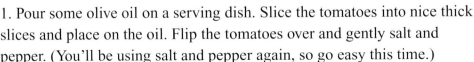

2. Fresh mozzarella cheese is sticky, so coat a sharp knife with olive oil prior to slicing cheese to prevent sticking. Slice the ball of cheese into ¼-inch-thick slices and layer with the tomato slices. Re-oil the knife if it starts to stick.

3. Finish with the basil, a sprinkling of olive oil, and salt and pepper to taste. Serve at room temperature.

TIP—Only prepare a tray large enough for 1 day. The tomatoes won't refrigerate well. This is also a great side dish with any meal.

Cream Cheese and Lox Rollups

Lox is thinly sliced salt-cured salmon. It can be found in your grocer's seafood section.

Ingredients	
6 ounces lox	
½ cup cream cheese (3.5 net carbs)	**9.5–11.5 Net Carbs for entire recipe**
1–2 tablespoons capers	
3–4 pieces GG Bran Crispbread (6–8 net carbs)	

1. Lay out each slice of lox individually.

2. Whip or fork-soften the cream cheese. Spread a layer on each lox slice, sprinkle capers on top of the cheese, and roll up the lox. Insert toothpicks through each rollup to make bite-size portions, and slice with a sharp knife.

3. Arrange the rollups on a snack tray and serve with GG Bran Crispbread.

Deli Rollups

Buy thinly sliced 0-carb meats and cheeses from your local deli for this snack tray.

Ingredients
Salt

5 asparagus spears (2 net carbs)
2 broccoli stalks (2 net carbs)
2 hearts of palm (1 net carb)
1 large sugar-free, zero-carb pickle
4 slices deli turkey breast
4 slices deli ham
4 slices deli roast beef
4 slices deli Cuban pork
4 slices deli Muenster cheese
4 slices deli American cheese
4 slices deli provolone cheese
4 slices deli Swiss cheese
16 pitted black olives (2 net carbs)
Extra-virgin olive oil
Freshly ground black pepper
Romano cheese, grated
Assorted 0-carb mustards

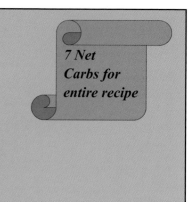

7 Net Carbs for entire recipe

1. Cook the asparagus and broccoli in a little salted water until cooked but not mushy. Cool the vegetables in cold water and pat dry. Cut the asparagus spears in half. Slice the broccoli, hearts of palm, and pickles in half lengthwise, then in half lengthwise again.

2. Lay out the meat slices on a serving tray and place the cheese slices on top, using 1 slice of cheese for each slice of meat.

3. Place half an asparagus spear on top of a cheese slice and roll up. Repeat with the broccoli, hearts of palm, and pickles, with 1 piece of vegetable per rollup.

4. Spear an olive with a toothpick and insert the toothpick through a rollup. Repeat for each rollup.

5. When you have made as many as you like, sprinkle each one with extra-virgin olive oil and a few grinds of pepper, and top with a sprinkling of Romano cheese.

6. Let the rollups rest at room temperature for 20 minutes before serving. Serve with a variety of 0-carb mustards.

Deviled Eggs

Ingredients
12 jumbo eggs (12 net carbs)
¼ cup mayonnaise
½ teaspoon dry mustard
Salt and pepper
Paprika
Fresh parsley leaves, finely chopped

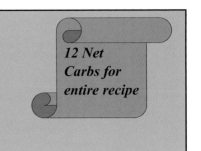

12 Net Carbs for entire recipe

1. Place the eggs in a saucepan in a single layer, and add cold water to cover by 2 inches. Cover the pot and bring to a boil over medium heat. As soon as the water starts to boil, remove the pan from the heat and let the eggs stand in hot water for 16 minutes.

2. Drain the hot water, then cover the eggs with cold water and ice cubes. Let stand until the eggs are completely cooled.

3. Peel the eggs under running water and pat dry. Slice the eggs in half lengthwise and remove the yolks. Place the yolks in a mixing bowl and arrange the sliced eggs on a serving platter.

4. To the yolks, add the mayonnaise, dry mustard, and salt and pepper to taste. Mix the yolks until smooth and spoon the mixture back into the eggs.

5. Sprinkle with paprika and parsley and refrigerate until ready to serve.

Beef Jerky

Ingredients
½ cup soy sauce (8 net carbs)
¼ cup Worcestershire sauce (11 net carbs)
¼ cup liquid smoke
¼ cup sugar-free teriyaki sauce
2 tablespoons stevia
2 tablespoons Cajun Land Cajun Seasoning

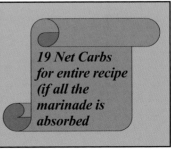

19 Net Carbs for entire recipe (if all the marinade is absorbed

4 pounds London broil (2 inches thick)
Red pepper flakes or freshly ground black pepper

1. For the marinade, mix together the soy sauce, Worcestershire sauce, liquid smoke, teriyaki sauce, stevia, and Cajun seasoning.

2. Slice the steak into ⅛-inch strips. Place the strips in the marinade, making sure to thoroughly coat each strip. Marinate for 48 hours, covered, in the refrigerator. Halfway through the process, mix the strips around in the bowl to redistribute the marinade, then return to the refrigerator and marinate for a second day.

3. Place the steak strips into a colander and drain all of the remaining marinade. Sprinkle red pepper flakes or grind black pepper to taste onto the strips and dry in a food dehydrator following the manufacturer's instructions.

TIP—I use Seal Sama Sugar-free Teriyaki Sauce, available at www.sealsama.com/teriyaki_sugar_free.html.

Video-supported recipe! Go to this Web site to watch me make it for you: www.FATtoSKINNY.com/recipes.htm.

Cajun Turnip Fries

Ingredients
¾ cup peanut oil
2 large turnips (6 net carbs)
1 tablespoon Cajun seasoning, such as Old Bay

6 Net Carbs for entire recipe

1. In a deep fryer, heat the peanut oil to 375 degrees.

2. Peel the turnips and cut them into pieces the size of french fries. Carefully add the turnips to the preheated oil and cook until golden brown and floating.

3. Remove the fries from the oil, drain well, and toss with the Cajun seasoning while the fries are still hot.

TIP—Replace the Cajun seasoning with any seasoning you like that complements the meal you are making. Just check the labels for carb counts.

Cheddar Cheese Crisps

Purchase your favorite sharp cheddar cheese for these crisps.

0 Net Carbs for entire recipe

Ingredients
12-ounce block of sharp cheddar cheese

1. Preheat the oven to 400 degrees.

2. Cut the cheddar into 1-inch cubes.

3. Line a cookie sheet with parchment paper and spread out 12 cheese cubes. Don't try to use foil; if you don't have parchment paper, spray non-stick cooking spray onto the cookie sheet.

4. Bake for 6 to 7 minutes, or until the cubes melt into flat crisps and are lightly brown around the edges.

5. Remove the crisps from the oven and let cool for 10 minutes before serving.

TIP—Like a little heat? Add fresh jalapeño slices to the tops of the cheese cubes before baking. You can also use shredded cheese mixed with various spices. Just roll the cheese and spices into balls (like meatballs) approximately 1 inch in diameter.

Jicama

I want to introduce you to jicama, a funny-looking vegetable. The cool thing about jicama is its very low carb count. Known as a "Mexican potato," jicama can be eaten raw or cooked. It's sweet and wonderful eaten raw in salads or cooked as you would home fries, hash browns, or French fries. It's crunchy raw and always retains a little crunch even when cooked. It's very low in starch and makes a great replacement for a traditional potato.

2.5 Net Carbs per ½ cup serving

You'll find it in the produce section of any quality grocer. When you see them at the store they should be very firm and dry. I suggest scratching a small piece of skin off at the store to make sure the jicama is white inside. If it's brown, chances are it will be brown all the way through and overripe. Fry in butter in a covered pan over medium heat, stirring often. Salt and pepper to taste and enjoy eating yourself skinny.

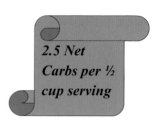

Video-supported recipe! Go to this Web site to watch me make it for you: **www.FATtoSKINNY.com/recipes.htm.**

Hot Capicola Jicama Wedges

Ingredients
½ small jicama, peeled (2.5 net carbs per ½ cup)
6 slices hot capicola (Italian cold cut)
1 tablespoon olive oil
1 tablespoon Balsamic Glaze (recipe below;
  6 net carbs)
Sea salt

8.5 Net Carbs for entire recipe

1. Slice the jicama into ⅛-inch-thick, half-moon slices.

2. Wrap the hot capicola around the jicama slices and arrange on a serving plate.

3. Drizzle olive oil and a tiny amount of Balsamic Glaze over the wedges. Sprinkle with sea salt to taste.

Balsamic Glaze—Over medium heat, reduce ½ cup of good balsamic vinegar to 50 percent volume, or until it reaches syrupy consistency.

TIP—Even though Balsamic Glaze is filled with carbs, a tiny amount adds the perfect sweetness that complements the hot capicola and brings out the apple undertones of the crisp jicama, so it's worth it for the negligible carbs added to the dish. Just be careful not to add too much.

Game Day Nachos

Each piece of Slim Trim Lavash has 11 carbs, but 10 are dietary fiber, so each whole flatbread is only 1 net carb. It is available at **www.samisbakery.com**.

Ingredients
2 Slim Trim Lavash (2 net carbs)
½ pound ground beef (or ground turkey, venison, or chicken)
1 teaspoon chili powder
1 teaspoon ground cumin
½ teaspoon cayenne pepper
1 teaspoon ground black pepper
1 teaspoon salt
½ cup shredded Mexican or cheddar cheese
2 tablespoons chopped onion (1.5 net carbs)
1 plum tomato, chopped (2.5 net carbs)
½ cup shredded lettuce (.5 net carb)
2 tablespoons sour cream (1 net carb)

7.5 Net Carbs for entire recipe

1. Lightly toast the lavash until the edges are golden brown.

2. Brown the ground meat in a skillet. Add the seasonings to the browned meat. Add cool water, 1 tablespoon at a time, until the desired thickness is reached, then set aside.

3. Break up the crispy lavash into chip-sized pieces. Place the chips on a cookie sheet, overlapping slightly. Add the meat to the chips and top with the shredded cheese. Place the cookie sheet under the broiler until the cheese is just melted, but not caramelized.

4. Remove from the oven and add the onion, tomato, lettuce, and a large dollop of sour cream.

 TIP—This can be a very filling snack because of the meat-to-chip ratio. Pile those lavash pieces with as much yummy topping as possible. If you like it spicy, add chopped jalapeños.

Avocado Zucchini Pillows

There is twice as much fiber in a Florida avocado than in its California brothers.

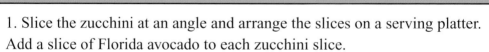

Ingredients
1 large Florida avocado (4 net carbs)
1 small zucchini (3 net carbs)
¼ cup sour cream (2.5 net carbs)
1 small jar Icelandic caviar (1 net carb
  per tablespoon)
1 tablespoon lemon juice (1 net carb)
Sea salt

13 Net Carbs for entire recipe

1. Slice the zucchini at an angle and arrange the slices on a serving platter. Add a slice of Florida avocado to each zucchini slice.

2. Drop a dollop of sour cream on top, then a dollop of caviar.

3. Sprinkle the lemon juice over the plate, sprinkle with sea salt to taste, and serve.

BREAKFAST

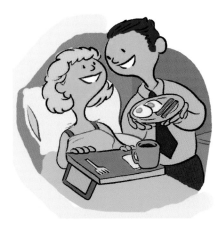

Scallion and Cheese Egg Beater Omelet with Baked Ham and Fresh Tomatoes

Use a nice slice of leftover baked ham for this hearty breakfast. Each cup of Egg Beaters egg substitute is equivalent to 4 whole eggs.

Ingredients
1 slice baked ham
2 teaspoons butter
2 tablespoons sour cream (1 net carb)
½ cup Egg Beaters (2 net carbs)
2 scallions, chopped (.5 net carbs)
¼ cup shredded cheddar cheese
½ small ripe tomato, sliced (1.5 net carbs)
Salt and pepper
1 piece GG Bran Crispbread (2 net carbs)

7 Net Carbs for entire recipe

1. Quickly pan-fry the ham in a little butter and set aside.

2. Over medium-low heat, melt 1 teaspoon butter in a nonstick skillet. Beat the sour cream into the egg product. Pour the eggs into the skillet and cover. Once the eggs start to set, top with the scallions and cheese and cover. Once the egg is completely set, fold the omelet in half and slip out of the pan onto a plate.

3. Arrange the tomato slices and the ham on the plate, salt and pepper to taste, and serve with GG Bran Crispbread.

TIP—Plan on having this breakfast the morning after your baked ham dinner (see page 198).

Raspberry Crepes

Crepes are very easy to make. They are simply very thin pancakes used to roll up a variety of ingredients.

Ingredients
1 large egg (1 net carb)
3 egg whites (1.5 net carbs)
1 tablespoon heavy cream
Sea salt
½ cup raspberries, plus additional for garnish (4 net carbs)
2 tablespoons sour cream (1.2 net carbs)
1 packet stevia
½ teaspoon lemon zest
2 tablespoons butter
Sugar-free whipped cream

8 Net Carbs for entire recipe

1. Add the egg, egg whites, cream, and a pinch of sea salt to a blender. Blend until incorporated and frothy.

2. Pour the mixture into a liquid measuring cup and place it in the refrigerator for 30 minutes. Rinse and dry the blender.

3. Add the raspberries, sour cream, stevia, and lemon zest to the blender, pulsing until all the ingredients are incorporated but not liquefied.

4. Over medium heat, melt a small pat of butter in a 6 to 8 inch nonstick crepe pan, swirling the melted butter to coat the pan. Add enough egg mixture to the pan to coat the bottom and up the sides of the pan while oscil-

lating your wrists to evenly distribute the mixture. Place the lid on the pan for *10 seconds* to firm the top of the crepe.

5. Slide the crepe onto a plate. Add a large spoonful of raspberry filling to the center of the crepe and then fold the sides over.

6. Repeat the process until you have made as many crepes as you desire (make sure to re-butter the pan when needed to prevent sticking).

7. Just before serving, add whipped cream and fresh berries for garnish.

TIP—You can substitute blackberries or strawberries for the raspberries, or try cream cheese, smoked salmon, and chives for a savory crepe.

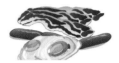

Fried Eggs with Smoked Sausage and "Home Fries"

Jicama stands in for high-sugar potatoes in this low-carb version of home fries. Unlike potatoes, jicama always retains a crunch. The trick to good eggs is cooking them over medium-low heat and with butter. I love my glass pan lids—they allow me to keep an eye on my eggs.

Ingredients
½ cup chopped jicama (2.5 net carbs)
2 tablespoons olive oil
2 teaspoons butter
2 jumbo eggs (2 net carbs)
1 smoked sausage link (1 net carb)
Salt and pepper
1 piece GG Bran Crispbread (2 net carbs)

7.5 Net Carbs for entire recipe

1. Peel the jicama and cut it into ½-inch slices, then stack those slices and cut into ½-inch strips. Turn the stack and cut into ½-inch cubes.

2. Heat 1 inch of lightly salted water in a skillet over high heat. Add the jicama cubes and cook until the water boils away. Keep an eye on the pan; the water will boil away fairly quickly. When the water is gone, mix in the olive oil. Stir well, cover, and reduce the heat to medium. Stir the jicama every few minutes to prevent burning. If it starts to burn, reduce the heat. Cook the jicama as if you're browning home fries. When the jicama presents a nice golden color, remove from the heat and stir in the butter. Remove the jicama from the pan and set it aside.

3. Cut the sausage lengthwise and fry it over medium heat, flat side down first, then flip it and cook the rounded side for a minute or two before removing it. Set aside.

4. Wipe out the skillet and return it to medium-low heat. Melt a pat of butter, spreading it around. Break the eggs into the pan and cook, covered, until the tops of the eggs are opaque.

5. Salt and pepper to taste. Serve the jicama, sausage, and eggs with GG Bran Crispbread.

Corned Beef Hash and Eggs

Use finely chopped leftover corned beef from a corned beef dinner, or open a can of corned beef. You can buy different brands at the store. Check the labels for carbs. Usually "hash" has potatoes, so stick with the can that says "100 percent corned beef."

Ingredients
1 can corned beef
2 jumbo eggs (2 net carbs)
Salt and pepper
2 pieces GG Bran Crispbread (4 net carbs)

6 Net Carbs for entire recipe

1. Put the corned beef into a nonstick frying pan and heat, covered, over medium heat until hot.

2. Hollow out 2 craters in the corned beef and break an egg into each crater.

3. Cover the pan and lower the heat to medium-low. Cook for 3 to 5 minutes, or until the tops of the eggs begin to look opaque.

4. Salt and pepper to taste. Serve with GG Bran Crispbread.

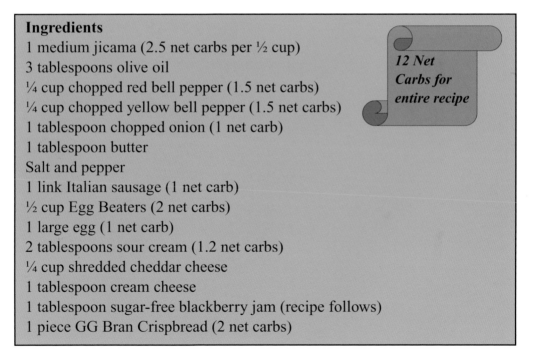

TIP—Plan on having this breakfast the morning after your corned beef and cabbage dinner (see page 200). My wife loves to sprinkle some shredded hot and spicy cheese (such as pepper jack) over the top during the last minute or two of cooking for an added "zing."

Cheddar Cheese Egg Beater Omelet "Surprise" with Italian Sausage and Jicama Roasted Pepper Medley

Ingredients
1 medium jicama (2.5 net carbs per ½ cup)
3 tablespoons olive oil
¼ cup chopped red bell pepper (1.5 net carbs)
¼ cup chopped yellow bell pepper (1.5 net carbs)
1 tablespoon chopped onion (1 net carb)
1 tablespoon butter
Salt and pepper
1 link Italian sausage (1 net carb)
½ cup Egg Beaters (2 net carbs)
1 large egg (1 net carb)
2 tablespoons sour cream (1.2 net carbs)
¼ cup shredded cheddar cheese
1 tablespoon cream cheese
1 tablespoon sugar-free blackberry jam (recipe follows)
1 piece GG Bran Crispbread (2 net carbs)

12 Net Carbs for entire recipe

1. Peel the jicama and cut it into ½-inch slices, then stack those slices and cut into ½-inch strips. Turn the stack and cut into ½-inch cubes.

2. Heat 1 inch of lightly salted water in a skillet over high heat. Add the jicama cubes and cook until the water boils away. Keep an eye on the pan; the water will boil away fairly quickly. When the water is gone, mix in 2 tablespoons olive oil, stir well, cover, and reduce the heat to medium. Stir the jicama every few minutes to prevent burning. If it starts to burn, reduce the heat. Cook the jicama as if you're browning home fries. Remember, unlike high-sugar potatoes, jicama always retains a crunch.

3. When the jicama presents a nice golden color, add the rest of the veggies and stir well. Continue cooking until all the veggies are softened to your liking. Remove the pan from the heat and stir in a couple pats of butter, then salt and pepper to taste. Remove the veggies to use as a side dish.

4. Place the skillet back on medium heat and add the remaining tablespoon of olive oil. Pierce the Italian sausage in a couple of places with a fork. Fry the sausage until golden brown, and then set aside.

5. Wipe out the skillet and return it to medium-low heat. Melt a pat of butter in the skillet. In a small bowl, combine the egg product and egg and beat the sour cream. Pour the eggs into the skillet and cover.

6. Now comes the "surprise": crack 1 egg in the middle of the omelet, being careful not to break the yolk. Once the egg starts to set, top with the cheddar cheese and cover. When the egg is completely set, fold the omelet in half and slip it out of the pan onto a plate.

7. Arrange the sausage and jicama on the plate and salt and pepper to taste. Serve with GG Bran Crispbread, cream cheese, and sugar-free blackberry jam.

Sugar-Free Blackberry Jam

Making sugar-free berry jam is easy. I recommend using blackberries, raspberries, and strawberries in my program and this easy recipe works for all of them (keep in mind that strawberries have a lower carb count than blueberries or raspberries).

Ingredients
2 cups fresh or frozen berries (16 net carbs)
8 packets stevia or ¼ cup xylitol

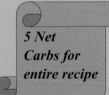

16 Net Carbs for entire recipe

1. Using a nonstick saucepan, cook down the berries over medium heat. (If you're using fresh berries, you'll need to add a little water to the saucepan.) You're looking for an "oatmeal" consistency. As you cook out the water and the berries start to thicken, stir often to avoid burning.

2. Once you've reached the proper consistency, remove the pan from the heat and immediately stir in the stevia or xylitol until the jam is sweet enough for your liking. The amount of sweetener needed will vary depending on your personal taste and the natural sweetness of the berries you're using.

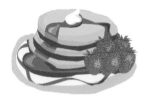

Strawberry Pancakes and Bacon

Ingredients
1 large egg (1 net carb)
1 tablespoon cream
2 tablespoons water (plus a little extra if needed)
2 teaspoons vanilla extract
3 tablespoons canola oil
½ cup NOW Foods Natural Almond Flour (2 net carbs)
1 teaspoon baking powder
1 tablespoon xylitol or 3 packets stevia
½ cup chopped fresh or frozen strawberries (2 net carbs)
8 strips Louis Rich turkey bacon or pork bacon
2 tablespoons butter
¼ cup Log Cabin Sugar-Free Syrup

5 Net Carbs for entire recipe

1. Heat a griddle or nonstick skillet over medium-high heat.

2. Beat the egg with the cream, water, vanilla, and 2 tablespoons canola oil. Add the almond flour, baking powder, and xylitol or stevia and mix well. Stir in the strawberries. Set aside and let the mixture stand while you cook the bacon.

3. Add 1 tablespoon of canola oil to the hot griddle or skillet. Fry the bacon until crisp, then set it aside.

4. Check the pancake batter for consistency—frozen strawberries are wetter than fresh strawberries and eggs come in different sizes, so you may have to adjust. Mix the batter with a spoon and see if it pours off the spoon in a semi-thick ribbon. If the batter is too thick, add 1 tablespoon of water at a time, mixing well and checking consistency as you go. If the batter is too watery, add 1 teaspoon of almond flour at a time, mixing well and checking consistency in between each addition.

5. Melt a tablespoon of butter and cook the pancakes, flipping once when the edges become golden brown. Re-butter the skillet or griddle in between batches.

6. Serve the pancakes topped with berries and syrup, with the bacon on the side.

TIP—Extra pancakes can be frozen or refrigerated. Heat them using a toaster oven.

Philly Cheese Steak and Egg Wraps

You can make this wrap with romaine lettuce or a La Tortilla Factory tortilla. I prefer to use the greens as wraps to keep the carb count at its lowest.

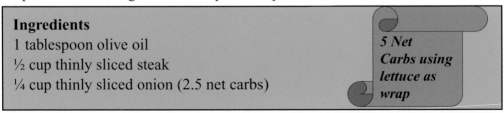

Ingredients
1 tablespoon olive oil
½ cup thinly sliced steak
¼ cup thinly sliced onion (2.5 net carbs)

5 Net Carbs using lettuce as wrap

2 large eggs (2 net carbs)
¼ cup shredded mozzarella cheese
1 romaine lettuce leaf (.5 net carbs) or La Tortilla Factory tortilla (3 net
   carbs)
Salt and pepper

1. Heat the olive oil in a nonstick skillet. Brown the steak and onion, then push to one side of the skillet. Scramble an egg in the pan, then mix the egg with the meat. Add the cheese and toss around to mix.

2. Drop the steak-and-egg mixture into a large romaine lettuce leaf. Salt and pepper to taste, then roll up the wrap and serve.

TIP—When slicing up steak for meat on a stick, slice extra and freeze in individual portion sizes for this meal.

Breakfast Pepperoni and Cheese Pizza

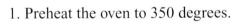

Ingredients
2 tablespoons olive oil
1 cup thinly sliced pepperoni
2 cups Egg Beaters (8 net carbs)
¾ cup shredded cheddar or mozzarella cheese
1 tablespoon grated Parmesan or Romano cheese
Salt and pepper

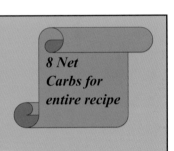

8 Net Carbs for entire recipe

1. Preheat the oven to 350 degrees.

2. Coat the bottom and sides of an ovenproof 10-inch skillet with olive oil. Line the skillet with the slices of pepperoni for the crust, reserving some for the top.

3. Slowly pour the egg product over the pepperoni crust, making sure the entire crust gets covered. The resulting pizza should be about ½ inch thick. Sprinkle the cheddar or mozzarella cheese on top of the eggs and place more pepperoni slices generously on top.

4. Bake for 25 minutes or until the eggs are set. To check if the eggs are set, gently press the center of the pizza—it should be firm to the touch.

5. Cut the pizza into slices. Sprinkle Parmesan or Romano cheese on top prior to serving.

TIP—To spice it up a bit, add chopped jalapeño peppers to the eggs. This dish works well served at room temperature. Make an extra pizza and cut it up for a snack tray.

Berry Berry Pecan Waffles with Ham

Serves 2

Ingredients
¼ cup New Hope Mills Sugar-Free Pancake and
   Waffle Mix (3 net carbs)
⅔ cup water
1 large egg (1 net carb)
¼ cup chopped pecans (1 net carb)
2 tablespoons vegetable oil
Nonstick cooking spray
Butter
½ cup blackberries and raspberries mixed (4 net carbs)
Sugar-free maple syrup
Sliced ham

9 Net Carbs for entire recipe

1. Beat the waffle mix with the water, oil, and egg until well mixed. Add the pecans to the batter and stir to incorporate.

2. Spray nonstick cooking spray on the waffle-maker surfaces and cook the waffles in your waffle maker according to the manufacturer's instructions.

3. Place a few fresh berries on each waffle and top with the syrup. Serve with a slice of ham left over from ham night.

TIP—Extra waffles can be frozen or refrigerated. Heat them using a toaster oven. Almost half the net carbs come from the berries. *Limit to once per week.*

Maple Sausage Egg Muffins

Ingredients

Nonstick cooking spray
2 large eggs (2 net carbs)
4 egg whites (2 net carbs)
2 teaspoons rubbed sage
4 packets stevia
1 teaspoon sugar-free maple extract
1 teaspoon sugar-free vanilla extract
Sea salt and fresh cracked black pepper
1 pound uncooked zero-carb breakfast sausage
12 1-inch cubes sharp cheddar cheese
Paprika

4 Net Carbs for entire recipe

1. Preheat the oven to 400 degrees.

2. Spray a 12-count muffin pan with nonstick cooking spray.

3. In a medium bowl, whisk together the eggs, egg whites, sage, stevia, maple extract, vanilla, a pinch of sea salt, and some pepper, then set aside.

4. Divide the sausage into 12 balls. Place a ball into the bottom of each muffin cup and press each one down to form a nice crust. Place a cheese cube in the center of each muffin cup, on top of the sausage. Ladle the egg mixture equally into the muffin cups

5. Bake for 20 minutes or until the egg completely sets and feels firm when touched in the center. Dust with paprika before serving.

—This muffin browns slightly and has a nice bread-like consistency. The eggs aren't as dense because of the high egg-white count. The sweetness and extracts make it taste like a maple syrup sausage, egg, and cheese biscuit. They freeze great, too, for a fast on-the-go breakfast.

Ham and Cheese Egg Beater Omelets with Sour Cream and Salsa

Ingredients
1 teaspoon butter
½ cup Egg Beaters (2 net carbs)
2 tablespoons plus 1 teaspoon sour cream (1.5 net carbs)
¼ cup chopped ham
¼ cup shredded cheddar cheese
2 tablespoons salsa (2 net carbs)
Salt and pepper
1 piece GG Bran Crispbread (2 net carbs)

7.5 Net Carbs for entire recipe

1. Melt the butter in a covered nonstick skillet over medium-low heat.

2. Beat 2 tablespoons sour cream into the egg product. Pour the eggs into the skillet and cover. Once the eggs start to set, top with the ham and cheese and cover.

3. Once the eggs are completely set, fold the omelet in half and slip it out of the pan onto a plate. Salt and pepper to taste. Spoon on the salsa and top with the remaining teaspoon sour cream. Serve with GG Bran Crispbread.

TIP—Plan on having this breakfast the morning after your baked ham dinner (see page 198).

Crepes Florentine

Ingredients

1 tablespoon butter, plus additional for crepe pan
2 tablespoons diced onion (1 net carb)
1 cup frozen spinach, thawed and chopped (2 net carbs)
½ teaspoon salt
¼ cup Bertolli Alfredo Sauce (3 net carbs)
2 large eggs (2 net carbs)
2 tablespoons New Hope Mills Sugar-Free Pancake and Waffle Mix (1.5 net carbs)
2 teaspoons water

9.5 Net Carbs for entire recipe

1. Heat a skillet over medium heat. Melt a teaspoon of butter in the skillet and quickly brown the onion. Add the spinach, salt, and half of the Alfredo sauce and mix well. Cook until the mixture is heated through, then cover and remove the pan from the stove.

2. Beat the eggs with the pancake mix and water; set aside.

3. Over medium heat, melt a small pat of butter in a small crepe pan, swirling the melted butter to coat the pan. Add enough batter to the pan to coat the bottom and up the sides of the pan while oscillating your wrists to evenly distribute the mixture. Place the lid on the pan for *45 seconds* to firm the top of the crepe.

4. Add a large spoonful of the spinach filling to the center of the crepe, fold the sides over in the pan, then slide the filled crepe onto a plate.

5. Repeat the process with the remaining batter and filling (make sure to re-butter the pan when needed to prevent sticking).

6. Serve the crepes drizzled with the remaining Alfredo sauce.

TIP—Make extra crepes and leave them in the fridge between paper towels for a dessert tonight. Fill with chopped strawberries and top with whipped cream for strawberry shortcake crepes. This recipe makes 4 8-inch crepes.

Crabmeat Omelet Alfredo

Ingredients
2 teaspoons butter
1 tablespoon diced onion (.5 net carb)
1 tablespoon diced bell pepper (.5 net carb)
1 clove garlic, minced (1 net carb)
4–6 ounces canned crabmeat
3 tablespoons Bertolli Alfredo sauce, room temperature (2.5 net carbs)
½ cup Egg Beaters (2 net carbs)
Salt and pepper

6.5 Net Carbs for entire recipe

1. Melt 1 teaspoon butter in a skillet over medium heat. Add the onion, bell pepper, and garlic, and sauté until soft. Stir in the crabmeat and 2 tablespoons of Alfredo sauce. Remove the filling to a side dish.

2. Wipe out the skillet and melt 1 teaspoon butter over medium heat. Pour in the Egg Beaters and cover. When the eggs are set on top, pour in the filling and fold over the omelet. Serve topped with the remaining Alfredo sauce. Salt and pepper to taste.

Lox and Cream Cheese with Capers and Red Onion

Ingredients
2 tablespoons cream cheese (1 net carb)
2 pieces GG Bran Crispbread (4 net carbs)
1 teaspoon capers
1 teaspoon minced red onion
4 ounces lox
Ground black pepper

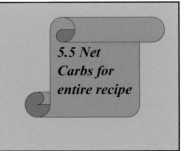

5.5 Net Carbs for entire recipe

1. Spread the cream cheese onto the GG Bran Crispbread.

2. Sprinkle the capers and red onion onto the cream cheese and top each piece with a slice of lox.

3. Grind some black pepper on top and serve.

Jicama Primavera

Ingredients
1 large jicama (7 net carbs)
2 tablespoons olive oil
½ cup chopped red bell pepper (3 net carbs)
½ cup chopped yellow bell pepper (3 net carbs)
¼ cup chopped onion (2.5 net carbs)
1 tablespoon butter
Salt and pepper

15.5 Net Carbs for entire recipe

1. Peel the jicama and cut it into ¾-inch cubes.

2. Heat 1 inch of lightly salted water in a skillet over high heat. Add jicama cubes and cook until the water boils away. Keep an eye on the pan; the water will boil away fairly quickly. As soon as the pan is dry, add the olive oil and the bell peppers and onion. Stir well, cover, and reduce the heat to medium.

3. Stir the jicama every few minutes to prevent burning. If it starts to burn, reduce the heat. Cook the jicama as if you're browning home fries. Remember, unlike high-sugar potatoes, jicama always retains a crunch.

4. Once all the veggies are softened to your liking, remove the pan from the heat and stir in the butter. Salt and pepper to taste and serve.

TIP—Cook plenty of jicama and leave it in the fridge for a fast heat-up in the microwave. I usually cook a couple jicama at a time, use what I need, and refrigerate the rest. It stores and reheats well when it's cooked.

Jicama turns bad quickly when stored uncooked, so it's best stored already cooked.

Eggs Smothered and Covered in a Jicama Basket with Turkey Bacon and Crispbread

Ingredients
6–8 slices turkey bacon
2 tablespoons butter
1 medium jicama (5 net carbs)
1 teaspoon olive oil
4 large eggs (4 net carbs)
2 tablespoons shredded cheddar cheese
2 pieces GG Bran Crispbread (4 net carbs)
Salt and pepper

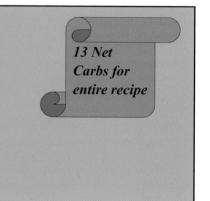

13 Net Carbs for entire recipe

1. In a medium skillet, pan-fry the turkey bacon in a tablespoon of butter until done to your likeness, then set it aside.

2. Peel the jicama and, using the largest holes of a handheld grater or a food processor, grate the jicama into hashbrowns. Rinse the shredded jicama under cold water, then strain and pat dry.

3. Heat the remaining butter and olive oil in a nonstick skillet over medium heat. Pan-fry the jicama for 5–6 minutes, or until it starts to brown around the edges.

4. Separate the jicama into two separate "baskets" and break 2 eggs into each basket. Cover and reduce the heat to medium-low.

5. Cook the eggs until the whites and the top of the yolk turn opaque. I like to use a glass cover on my skillet so I can keep an eye on things.

6. Sprinkle the cheese on top, cover, and turn off the heat. While the cheese melts, arrange the bacon and GG Bran Crispbread on plates. Gently scoop out the baskets and serve. Salt and pepper to taste.

Denver Egg Beater Omelet

Ingredients

1 tablespoon butter
¼ cup chopped ham
2 tablespoons chopped red bell pepper (.75 net carb)
2 tablespoons chopped green bell pepper (.75 net carb)
1 tablespoon diced onion (.5 net carb)
½ cup Egg Beaters (2 net carbs)
Fresh parsley sprigs, for garnish
Salt and pepper

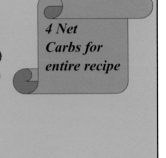

4 Net Carbs for entire recipe

1. Over medium-low heat, melt some butter in a covered nonstick skillet, then toss in the ham, bell peppers, and onion. Stir-fry until the onion starts to soften. Remove 1 tablespoon of the mixture and set aside for a topping.

2. Pour the Egg Beaters into the skillet, mix gently, and cover. Once the egg is completely set, fold the omelet in half and slip it out of the pan onto a plate.

3. Top with the reserved ham, peppers, and onion. Garnish with parsley and season with salt and pepper to taste.

Blueberry Pancakes

Ingredients

¼ cup New Hope Mills Sugar-free Pancake and
   Waffle Mix (3 net carbs)
⅔ cup water
1 large egg (1 net carb)
2 tablespoons vegetable oil
1 teaspoon vanilla extract
2 tablespoons fresh or frozen blueberries (2.5 net carbs)
1 tablespoon butter
Log Cabin Sugar-Free Syrup

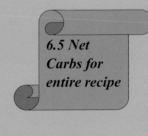

6.5 Net Carbs for entire recipe

1. Preheat the oven to 225 degrees.

2. Beat the pancake mix with the water, egg, oil, and vanilla in a medium bowl. Add the chopped blueberries to the batter and stir to combine.

3. Cook the pancakes on a hot buttered griddle.

4. Serve with Log Cabin Sugar Free syrup.

TIP—Extra pancakes can be frozen or refrigerated. Reheat in a toaster oven. *Limit to once per week.*

Steak and Eggs

Ingredients
1 teaspoon butter
2 large eggs (2 net carbs)
4–6 ounces sliced steak
Fresh parsley sprigs, for garnish
2 pieces GG Bran Crispbread (4 net carbs)
1–2 tablespoons cream cheese (1 net carb)
Salt and pepper

5 Net Carbs for entire recipe

1. Melt the butter in a nonstick skillet over medium-low heat. Gently crack and drop in the eggs and cover the pan. I prefer to use a glass lid so I can watch my eggs. When the eggs reach an opaque color, slide them onto a plate.

2. Raise the heat to medium-high and quickly pan-fry the steak slices to your preferred doneness. Slide the steak onto the plate with the eggs.

3. Salt and pepper to taste, garnish with parsley, and serve with GG Bran Crispbread and cream cheese.

TIP—I like to freeze packets of sliced steak in individual servings when I'm cutting London broil for beef jerky (see page 133). Simply buy an extra steak, slice it up, and place 4 or 5 slices into small freezer bags for a quick breakfast, brunch, or Philly cheese steak wrap (see page 192).

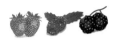

Fresh Fruit and Cream

Yum yum, who says you can't enjoy fresh fruit on a low-sugar, low-carb diet? I recommend strawberries, blackberries, and raspberries as part of the FAT TO SKINNY eating plan. I allow kiwi in smaller quantities to bring in the banana flavor. Keep the total per-serving quantity to 1 cup. This makes a delicious, light breakfast, snack, or dessert.

Ingredients
¼ cup strawberries (1 net carb)
¼ cup blackberries (2 net carbs)
¼ cup raspberries (2 net carbs)
2 tablespoons kiwi (3 net carbs)
¼ cup ice-cold heavy cream

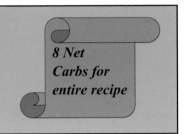

8 Net Carbs for entire recipe

1. Combine the fruit in a bowl.

2. Pour on the cream and serve immediately.

TIP—While you're cleaning and cutting the fruit, make some sugar-free Jell-O or mousse for dessert.

Fall Frittata with Fresh Tomato, Scallions, and Romano Cheese

Buy Miracle Noodles at **www.miraclenoodle.com**. They are a wonderful, completely **SUGAR**-free product to replace traditional pasta.

Ingredients
1 package Miracle Noodles angel hair pasta
Salt and pepper

1 tablespoon butter
2 large eggs (2 net carbs)
2 tablespoons shredded cheddar cheese
½ small ripe tomato, chopped (1.5 net carbs)
2 scallions, chopped (.5 net carbs)
1 tablespoon grated Romano cheese

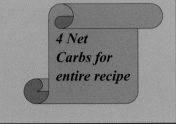

4 Net Carbs for entire recipe

1. Open the package of noodles. They are already cooked, so simply drop them in a strainer and rinse well.

2. While the noodles are draining, melt the butter in a nonstick skillet over medium heat.

3. Beat the eggs well in a medium bowl. Pat the noodles dry with a paper towel and mix in with the eggs and a little salt and pepper.

4. When the butter is sizzling, pour the eggs and pasta into the pan and cover.

5. When the edges of the frittata are well set, flip it over with a spatula, sprinkle the cheddar cheese on top, and cover. Continue cooking for another 2 to 3 minutes.

6. Slide the frittata onto a plate and sprinkle the tomato, scallions, and Romano cheese on top. Season with salt and pepper to taste, and serve.

TIP—Rinse the noodles well. The liquid they come in has a bit of a fishy smell you'll want to rinse out. For this recipe, make sure to pat the noodles dry after rinsing.

LUNCH

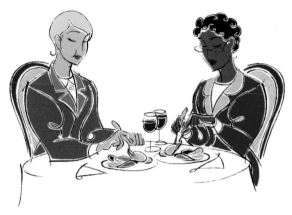

Tuna Wrap with Black Olives and Jalapeño

Ingredients
1 can tuna
3 tablespoons mayonnaise
7 pitted medium black olives, chopped (1 net carb)
1 jalapeño pepper, chopped
1 romaine lettuce leaf (.5 net carbs) or La Tortilla
  Factory tortilla (3 net carbs)
Salt and pepper
Fried pork rinds
1 large dill pickle (2 net carbs)

6 Net Carbs for entire recipe

1. Mix the tuna with your favorite carb-free mayonnaise. Add the olives and jalapeño.

2. Place the tuna salad in a large romaine lettuce leaf, season with salt and pepper to taste, then roll up the wrap. If you prefer, you can substitute a La Tortilla Factory tortilla for the romaine. I prefer the greens as wraps to keep the meal 100 percent SUGAR-free.

3. Serve with fried pork skins and a dill pickle.

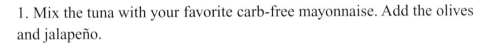

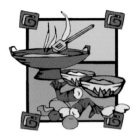

TIP—Wraps can be made from the leftovers in your fridge or from the wide variety of meats and cheeses available from your deli. When buying sliced lunch meat, make sure to stay away from any meats cured with SUGAR or honey. CHECK THE LABELS.

Oriental Stir-Fry Veggies

Seal Sama Sugar-Free Teriyaki Sauce is available from **www.sealsama.com**.

Ingredients
2 tablespoons Seal Sama Sugar-Free Teriyaki Sauce
1 tablespoon soy sauce (1 net carb)
1 tablespoon olive oil
1 tablespoon sesame oil
1 clove garlic, finely chopped (1 net carb)
1 tablespoon finely chopped fresh ginger (1 net carbs)
1 cup shredded green cabbage (3 net carbs)
½ cup chopped bok choy, including the green leafy tops (.5 net carbs)
¼ cup sliced red bell pepper (1.5 net carbs)
¼ cup sliced yellow bell pepper (1.5 net carbs)
¼ cup sliced onion (2.5 net carbs)
Salt and pepper

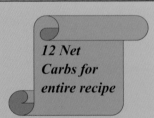

12 Net Carbs for entire recipe

1. Mix the teriyaki sauce with the soy sauce and set aside.

2. Now it's time to cook. Heat the olive oil and sesame oil in a large skillet or wok over high heat. At the first sign of smoke, toss in the garlic and ginger first, then all the remaining chopped veggies. Count to 10, then stir-fry the ingredients in the pan.

3. As soon as the cabbage starts to show the first signs of wilting, pour in the sauce and continue to stir-fry for another couple of minutes. Serve immediately. Salt and pepper to taste.

TIP—While you have the veggies out, cut extra, bag them together and store in the fridge for another quick stir-fry. Use within two days to prevent browning. For a hearty variation to this meal, you can add shrimp, small chunks of chicken breast, or beef. To cook, stir-fry any of those proteins first, then add the garlic and ginger, then the vegetables.

Italian Chef's Salad with Radicchio and Walnuts

Ingredients
1½ cups mixed lettuces (1.5 net carbs)
¼ cup radicchio (.5 net carb)
3 slices prosciutto
3 slices Genoa salami
3 slices mortadella
3 slices provolone cheese
5 green olives, pitted (2.5 net carbs)
1 hardboiled egg, halved (1 net carb)
1 tablespoon chopped walnuts (.5 net carb)
2 tablespoons extra-virgin olive oil
1 tablespoon red wine vinegar
Salt and pepper

6 Net Carbs for entire recipe

1. Prepare a bed of your favorite lettuces, including radicchio in the mix.

2. Roll up slices of the prosciutto, Genoa salami, mortadella, and provolone cheese and place on the greens. Add the olives and hardboiled egg. Salt and pepper to taste. Sprinkle walnuts on top.

3. Dress with the olive oil and red wine vinegar and serve.

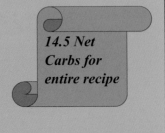

TIP—While you have the greens out, prepare some side salads in bowls that you can leave covered with plastic wrap in the fridge. While the meat and cheese are out, make some rollups for a snack tray.

Deep-Fried Shrimp with Sweet and Hot Wasabi Jicama Coleslaw

Ingredients
1½ cups shredded green cabbage (4.5 net carbs)
1 cup shredded purple cabbage (3 net carbs)
½ cup finely julienned jicama (2.5 net carbs)
Salt and pepper
3 tablespoons Kraft Green Goddess Dressing (3 net carbs)
1 tablespoon wasabi mustard (mixed from powder or paste)
1 tablespoon sour cream (.5 net carb)
1 tablespoon mayonnaise
1 teaspoon stevia
1 large egg (1 net carb)
2 tablespoons heavy cream
8–12 large shrimp, cleaned and deveined
1 cup Fry Coating (see page 251)
1½ cups peanut oil
3 tablespoons sugar-free ketchup
1 teaspoon prepared horseradish

14.5 Net Carbs for entire recipe

1. Place the cabbage and jicama in a mixing bowl and salt and pepper to taste.

2. In a separate bowl, mix the green goddess dressing, wasabi, sour cream, mayonnaise, and stevia.

3. Add the dressing to the vegetables and mix well, then set aside.

4. Beat the egg with the cream in a medium bowl and place the shrimp in the egg wash. Mix the shrimp around with your fingers to make sure they all get a good coating, then dredge the shrimp in the Fry Coating. Using a

deep fryer or a deep skillet, deep fry the shrimp in 375-degree peanut oil 2 to 3 minutes per side, or until golden brown.

5. Mix the ketchup and horseradish together and serve this homemade cocktail sauce with the shrimp and coleslaw.

TIP—Process extra pork rinds from the Fry Coating in a food processor and store the ground Fry Coating in a zippered plastic bag in the pantry. The coating works well for all fried foods, including fish and chicken. The coleslaw is very good the next day, too, if you wish to make a double batch. Typical deep-fry temperatures range between 325 and 400 degrees. The shrimp in this recipe are best cooked at 375 degrees.

Wasabi Spinach Salad

I like the Tsunami brand wasabi products, available in many grocers' seafood departments or at the following Web site: **www.afcsushi.com**.

Ingredients
1½ cups fresh spinach (1 net carb)
3 tablespoons roughly chopped walnuts (1.5 net carbs)
2 scallions, roughly chopped (.5 net carb)
1 tablespoon Tsunami wasabi dressing (1 net carb)

4 Net Carbs for entire recipe

Clean the spinach and pat it dry. In a salad bowl, combine the spinach with the walnuts and scallions. Toss with the wasabi dressing and serve.

Eggs in a Portobello Nest

Ingredients
1 teaspoon butter
2 large portobello mushrooms (3 net carbs)
4 tablespoons chopped ham
2 large eggs (2 net carbs)

5 Net Carbs for entire recipe

2 tablespoons grated Romano cheese
Cracked pepper

1. Select a large frying pan with a form-fitting lid, preferably a see-through lid. Heat the butter in the pan over medium heat.

2. Remove the stems from the mushrooms and rinse the caps clean under the faucet. Add 2 tablespoons of the chopped ham to the cavity of each mushroom. Place the mushroom caps into the melted, sputtering butter, ham side up.

3. Crack each egg and carefully pour the egg over the ham until the mushroom caps are full but not flowing over the edges. Place the lid on the pan and steam until the egg whites become opaque.

4. Remove the lid and sprinkle a tablespoon of Romano over the tops. Cover the pan and cook another 60 seconds or until the cheese melts.

5. Remove the mushrooms from the pan to a serving plate. Add fresh cracked pepper to taste.

Crab Salad–Stuffed Avocados

Ingredients
1 cup shredded iceberg lettuce (1 net carb)
½ Florida avocado (2 net carbs)
1 tablespoon key lime juice (1 net carb)
¾ cup lump crabmeat
1 tablespoon mayonnaise
Sea salt
Cracked black pepper or Caribbean pepper

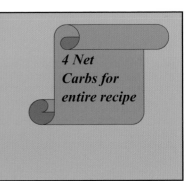

4 Net Carbs for entire recipe

1. Prepare a bed of lettuce on a lunch-sized plate.

2. Cut the avocado by running a sharp knife into the fruit until it hits the seed.

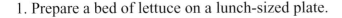

Cut a line lengthwise around the circumference of the avocado. Now, with your hands, twist the fruit until it separates in half. Rest the avocado half, cut side up, on the bed of lettuce. Sprinkle lime juice over the avocado and lettuce.

3. Fold together the crabmeat and mayonnaise in a small bowl. Salt to taste.

4. Use an ice cream scoop to scoop out the crab mixture and place it in the avocado void. Crack black or Caribbean pepper over the dish to taste, and enjoy.

 TIP—A can of drained tuna works well, too, if crab isn't available.

Grilled Cheeseburger and Chips

Top a burger with your favorite cheese (try smoked Gouda for a change) and serve in a romaine lettuce wrap instead of a bun. If you prefer, you can substitute La Tortilla Factory tortillas for the lettuce. I prefer the greens as wraps to keep the burger as SUGAR-free as possible.

Ingredients
¼ pound ground beef
1 slice cheese
1 slice onion (.75 net carb)
1 slice ripe tomato (.5 net carb)
1 romaine lettuce leaf (.5 net carbs) or La Tortilla
  Factory tortilla (3 net carbs)
Pork rinds (0 net carbs) or EatSmart Soy Crisps (3 net carbs per 10 chips)
1 large sugar-free dill pickle (2 net carbs)

3.75 Net Carbs for entire recipe using lettuce and pork rinds

1. Grill that burger any way you like it, top with the cheese, and cut in half.

2. Wrap it in the lettuce leaf with the onion and tomato.

3. Serve with pork rinds or a measured amount of EatSmart Soy Crisps and a big dill pickle (SUGAR-free, of course).

Mexican Taco Salad

Ingredients
1 tablespoon olive oil
¼ pound ground beef
2 tablespoons diced onion (1 net carb)
1 big clove garlic, chopped (1 net carb)
1 tablespoon chopped jalapeño pepper (.5 net carb)
¼ teaspoon ground cumin
Salt and pepper
2 cups mixed lettuces (2 net carbs)
10 EatSmart Soy Crisps (3 net carbs)
¼ cup shredded cheddar cheese

7.5 Net Carbs for entire recipe

1. Heat up the olive oil in a skillet. Pan-fry the ground beef with the onion, garlic, jalapeño, cumin, and salt and pepper to taste. Continue cooking until no red color is visible in the beef and the onions have softened. When it is cooked, drain the meat in a strainer.

2. Fill a bowl with your favorite salad mix. Place EatSmart Soy Crisps around the rim of the bowl. Spoon a generous amount of the meat mixture on top while still hot and sprinkle with cheese. Serve immediately.

TIP—Plan this lunch the day after your cheeseburgers to use up ground beef in the fridge.

Fettuccini Alfredo Primavera

This is a wonderful, fast lunch that can be prepared in advance and taken to work or quickly put together at work in a microwave.

Ingredients
1 package Tofu Shirataki Fettuccini (2 net carbs)
¼ cup roughly chopped yellow bell pepper (1.5 net carbs)
¼ cup roughly chopped zucchini (.75 net carb)

¼ cup roughly chopped broccoli (1 net carb)
¼ cup roughly chopped mushrooms (1 net carb)
¼ cup grated Parmesan or Romano cheese
½ cup Rich and Creamy Alfredo Sauce, recipe follows
   (.5 net carb)
Salt and pepper
1 tablespoon chopped fresh basil

6.75 Net Carbs for entire recipe

1. Strain the noodles and rinse well. Mix the noodles with the veggies in a bowl. Top with a good sprinkling of grated cheese and the Alfredo sauce.

2. Place the bowl in the microwave and heat through, mixing once halfway through process.

3. Top with more grated cheese, salt and pepper to taste, and some chopped basil, then serve.

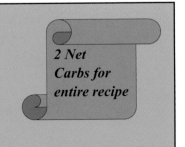

TIP—This recipe holds up very well. The pasta doesn't get mushy like traditional wheat pasta, so you can make a couple of servings in advance and store in the fridge at work for a quick, hot lunch.

Video-supported recipe! Go to this Web site to watch me make it for you: **www.FATtoSKINNY.com/recipes.htm**.

Rich and Creamy Alfredo Sauce

Makes 2.5 cups

Ingredients
¼ cup salted butter
1 cup heavy cream
1 clove garlic, crushed (1 net carb)
1½ cups grated Parmesan cheese
1 tablespoon chopped fresh parsley (1 net carb)
1 teaspoon cracked black pepper

2 Net Carbs for entire recipe

Melt the butter in a saucepan over medium-low heat. Sauté the garlic in the butter for 1 minute. Whisk in the cream and simmer for 5 minutes or until hot enough to melt the cheese. Add the cheese and whisk quickly, making sure to melt the cheese completely. Stir in the parsley and pepper and serve.

TIP—Substitute this sauce for any recipe calling for Alfredo sauce. Many recipes in this book call for Bertolli Alfredo sauce from a jar. Although this cuts down on prep time, it increases carbs 3 net grams per ¼ cup. Using the above recipe will cut down total net carb count substantially.

Jamaican Jerk Chicken with Strawberry Sauce

Serves 2

These chicken breasts get their kick from Jamaican jerk seasoning. Whichever you use, check the label for SUGAR. My personal favorite is the Walkerswood brand; it's most likely at your supermarket, and can be found at **www.walkerswood.com**. It's 1 net carb per teaspoon, but you lose half the seasoning on the grill surface.

Ingredients
2 boneless, skinless chicken breasts
2 tablespoons Jamaican jerk seasoning (3 net carbs)
¾ cup strawberries, trimmed and chopped (3 net carbs)
¼ cup crushed ice
2 large whole romaine lettuce leaves (1 net carb)
Salt and pepper

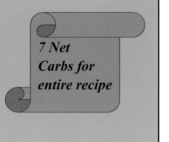
7 Net Carbs for entire recipe

1. Heat up the grill. Using a sharp knife, cut five or six ¼-inch-deep slits across each chicken breast. Rub the breasts with dry or wet Jamaican jerk seasoning and salt and pepper to taste. Place the breasts on the hot grill.

2. While the chicken is grilling, put the strawberries in a blender with the ice and puree into a nice sauce.

3. Arrange a bed of lettuce on two plates and pour a generous amount of strawberry sauce in the middle of each, reserving a few tablespoons for a topping.

4. Slice each breast on an angle and fan across the sauce. Decorate the top with the reserved sauce and serve.

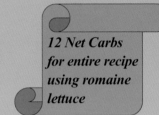 **TIP**—Cook extra breasts for a snack tray, cut in strips, and serve at room temperature. Dip into cold strawberry sauce.

Steak and Chicken Fajitas with Spicy Avocado Spread

Serves 2

Ingredients
½ pound steak
1 large boneless, skinless chicken breast
½ cup sliced onion (5 net carbs)
½ cup sliced bell pepper (3 net carbs)
1 tablespoon ground cumin
Salt and pepper
½ cup Florida avocado (2 net carbs)
2 tablespoons sour cream (1 net carbs)
1 teaspoon cayenne pepper (more for hot, less for mild)
1 tablespoon olive oil
2 large romaine lettuce leaves (.5 net carbs each) or 2 La Tortilla Factory
   tortillas (3 net carbs each)
½ cup shredded cheddar cheese

12 Net Carbs for entire recipe using romaine lettuce

1. Cut the steak and chicken into thin strips.

2. Season the meat, onion, and bell pepper with the cumin and salt and pepper to taste. Set aside.

3. Scoop the avocado into a bowl and add the sour cream and ground red pepper. Mash the fruit into a paste, and add salt and pepper to taste.

4. Heat the olive oil in a cast iron skillet over high heat. When the oil begins to smoke, quickly stir-fry the meats and veggies together until the chicken is cooked through.

5. Place the steaming hot skillet on a trivet in the center of the table. Arrange a plate of large romaine lettuce leaves to be used as wraps. If you prefer, you can substitute La Tortilla Factory tortillas for the romaine lettuce. I prefer the greens as wraps to keep the meal as SUGAR-free as possible.

6. Serve with the cheese and avocado spread.

 TIP—Cook extra chicken, steak, and veggies for salad toppings.

Fajita Salad

Using the recipe above, omit the avocado spread and wraps. Place a serving of warm meat and vegetables on top of 1 cup green salad per person. This has 5.5 Net Carbs per serving.

Steamed Artichokes with Roasted Garlic, Avocado and Lemon Dipping Sauce

Serves 2

Ingredients
2 fresh artichokes (14 net carbs)
½ cup chicken broth
2 teaspoons olive oil
5 cloves garlic, crushed (5 net carbs)
1 large Florida avocado (4 net carbs)
2 tablespoons lemon juice (2 net carbs)
Sea salt and cracked black pepper

25 Net Carbs for entire recipe

1. Rinse the artichokes under running water and trim the spikes off each leaf with kitchen shears.

2. Add the artichokes and chicken broth to a pressure cooker. Bring the

pressure up to temperature and cook for 15 minutes. Release the pressure and set aside to cool slightly.

3. Heat a small pan over medium heat and add the olive oil. Add the garlic to the heated oil and cook, slowly reducing the heat to medium-low and stirring constantly until the garlic is golden brown and smells nutty.

4. Combine the avocado, lemon juice, garlic, and salt and pepper to taste in a food processor. Blend well until creamy.

5. Serve the artichokes with the avocado sauce on the side.

TIP—If you do not have a pressure cooker, you can steam the artichokes in the oven. Place the artichokes in a covered baking dish with 1 inch of water in the bottom. Bake at 375 degrees for 45 minutes. This is a fairly high-carb lunch, so plan it on a day when all your other food choices are very low-carb.

Open-Faced Pesto Quesadilla

Use a toaster oven to make this dish for a quick meal. Note the back of the package of Slim Trim Lavash: each piece has 11 carbs, but 10 are dietary fiber, so 1 whole flatbread is only 2 net carbs. It is available at **www.samisbakery.com**.

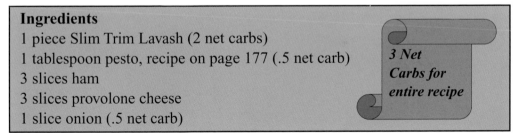

Ingredients
1 piece Slim Trim Lavash (2 net carbs)
1 tablespoon pesto, recipe on page 177 (.5 net carb)
3 slices ham
3 slices provolone cheese
1 slice onion (.5 net carb)

3 Net Carbs for entire recipe

1. Spread the lavash with a thin layer of pesto. Layer 2 slices of ham on the pesto, then cut another ham slice in half and fill in the empty areas. Do the same thing with the provolone cheese. Sprinkle the onion evenly on top of the cheese.

2. Toast for 10 minutes or until the crust is golden brown and the cheese starts to caramelize.

TIP—If you don't have a toaster oven you can still make this recipe with ease. Preheat the oven to 400 degrees and bake the quesadilla following the instructions above for 10 minutes, preferably on a pizza stone you preheated in the oven.

Grilled Chicken-Eggplant Sandwiches

Serves 2

Ingredients
1 medium eggplant (8 net carbs)
¾ cup shredded cooked chicken breast
1 small celery stalk, finely chopped (.5 net carb)
2 tablespoons mayonnaise
1 tablespoon diced onion (.5 net carb)
Salt and pepper
Nonstick cooking spray
4 slices provolone cheese

11 Net Carbs for entire recipe

1. Cut the eggplant at an angle into four ¼-inch-thick slices.

2. In a small bowl, combine the chicken, celery, mayonnaise, onion, and salt and pepper to taste. Mix all the ingredients very well, being sure to shred the chicken into fine pieces, leaving no large clumps.

3. Spray a heated sandwich press with enough nonstick cooking spray to coat both sides thoroughly. Place the eggplant on the press and trim if necessary. (The eggplant acts as the "bread" for the sandwich.)

4. Spoon the chicken salad into the center of the eggplant and top with two slices of cheese, completing the sandwich with another slice of eggplant. Press togeth-

er on high heat until the eggplant is a golden brown. Remove the cooked sandwich and plate. Repeat with the remaining ingredients for a second sandwich.

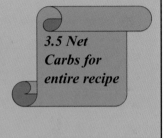 **TIP**—Liquid is going to be your enemy in this dish, so drain the chicken extremely well if using canned chicken and don't overdo the mayo.

Chicken Pecan Salad

This is an easy recipe to make after any baked chicken meal. It can be served inside a wrap or simply scooped on top of your favorite green salad mix, as we do here.

Ingredients
1 cup chopped cooked chicken
2 tablespoons diced scallions or red onion (1 net carb)
2 tablespoons roughly chopped pecans (.5 net carb)
¼ cup mayonnaise
Salt and pepper
2 cups mixed lettuces (2 net carbs)

3.5 Net Carbs for entire recipe

1. Combine the chicken with the scallions or onion, pecans, and mayonnaise in a small bowl.

2. Salt and pepper the salad to taste.

3. Prepare a bed of your favorite lettuces, scoop the chicken salad on top, and serve.

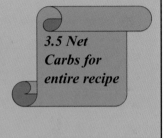 **TIP**—This is a great salad to stuff into avocado halves. Spritz the avocado with sweet lemon spray to give extra flavor to the dish as well as slow browning of the avocado. Simply mix 2 tablespoons lemon juice with 2 tablespoons water and 1 or 2 packets stevia (depending on desired sweetness) and mix well. Pour the mixture into a spray bottle and spritz the stuffed avocados.

Cajun Seafood Salad

I make this wonderful salad the day after we have a Cajun seafood boil (recipe on page 201). This is best served over a green salad or as a wrap in a La Tortilla Factory tortilla or a romaine lettuce leaf. You can also serve as a spread using GG Bran Crispbread.

Ingredients
1 cup leftover Cajun fish and shrimp
2 tablespoons chopped scallions or red onion (1 net carb)
¼ cup mayonnaise
Salt and pepper

1 Net Carbs for entire recipe

Chop the leftover fish and shrimp from the boil and place into a mixing bowl. Add the scallions or red onion and mayonnaise and mix well. Salt and pepper to taste, then serve.

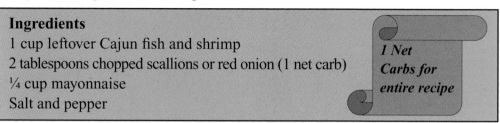

TIP—If you don't have leftovers from a seafood boil, substitute canned tuna spiced up with Cajun Land Cajun Seasoning.

Italian Sausage, Onion, and Pepper Wraps

Serves 4

Ingredients
1 tablespoon olive oil
4 Italian sausage links (4 net carbs)
½ cup sliced onion (5 net carbs)
½ cup sliced bell pepper (3 net carbs)
Salt and pepper
4 large romaine lettuce leaves (.5 net carbs each)
   or 4 La Tortilla Factory tortillas (3 net carbs each)

12.5 Net Carbs for entire recipe using lettuce

1. Heat the olive oil in a skillet over medium heat. Add the sausage and cook until browned and cooked through. Add the onion and bell pepper to the pan and cover. Cook until vegetables soften. Salt and pepper to taste.

2. Serve the sausages, peppers, and onions wrapped in large romaine lettuce leaves. If you prefer, you can substitute La Tortilla Factory tortillas for the romaine lettuce, but I prefer the greens as wraps to keep the meal as SUGAR-free as possible.

 TIP—Cook extra sausages and cut them into 1-inch pieces. Stick a toothpick in each one and place in the fridge for a snack tray. Reheat gently in the microwave before serving. I find most prepackaged Italian sausage is 1 carb per link. Order fresh sausage from your local butcher made with 100 percent meat and your sausage will be carb-free.

Wilted Spinach and Bacon Salad

Ingredients
1 cup fresh spinach, packed (1 net carb)
2 slices cooked bacon, roughly chopped
1 tablespoon olive oil
1 tablespoon lemon juice (1 net carb)
1 packet stevia
1 piece GG Bran Crispbread (2 carbs)

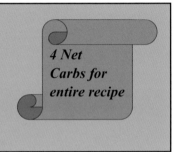

4 Net Carbs for entire recipe

1. Wash the spinach and pat it dry. Place it in a mixing bowl and add the bacon.

2. Mix a dressing using the olive oil and lemon juice. Sweeten the dressing with stevia until it reaches the desired sweetness. Heat the dressing in the microwave until it becomes very warm but not boiling.

3. Mix the dressing into the salad and toss. Serve with GG Bran Crispbread.

Lump Crab Cakes with Sherry Pesto

Ingredients
1 tablespoon mayonnaise

1 large egg (1 net carb)
1 teaspoon lemon or orange zest (1 net carb)
½ teaspoon cayenne pepper
1 cup lump crabmeat
¼ cup olive oil
Salt and pepper

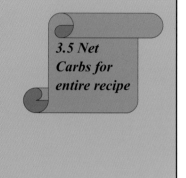

3.5 Net Carbs for entire recipe

Sherry Pesto
2 tablespoons sour cream (1 net carb)
1 tablespoon extra dry sherry
1 tablespoon pesto, recipe follows (.5 net carb)

1. In a large mixing bowl, whip together the mayonnaise, egg, zest, salt and pepper, and cayenne, adding additional cayenne to taste for your desired heat level. Once the creamed sauce is well incorporated with a whisk, fold in the crabmeat, being careful not to break up the lump pieces too much; set aside.

2. In a separate bowl, whisk together the sour cream, sherry, and pesto, to make the Pesto Sherry Cream Sauce.

3. Heat a cast iron skillet with enough olive oil to coat the pan, starting at high heat and reducing the heat to medium just before the oil smokes. Spoon out the crab cake mixture into 4 cakes. Shape the mixture into rounds using a spatula. Cook until the cakes firm and are golden brown, then flip carefully.

4. Serve with a spoonful of Pesto Sherry Cream Sauce.

TIP—Make this recipe an appetizer! Substitute the cast iron skillet with a mini-muffin pan. Spray the pan liberally with a nonstick cooking spray and drop spoonfuls of crab into each muffin cup. You can even add grated hard Italian cheese to the tops for an extra kick. Bake in a preheated 400-degree oven for 20 minutes. Pop the crab cakes out of the muffin cups, place them into a decorative bowl, and serve with the Pesto Sherry Cream Sauce.

Pesto

Makes 1 cup

Ingredients
2 cups fresh basil leaves, packed (3 net carbs)
½ cup extra-virgin olive oil
⅓ cup chopped pine nuts or walnuts (3 net carbs)
3 large garlic cloves, minced (3 net carbs)
½ cup grated Parmesan or Romano cheese
¼ teaspoon salt
Freshly ground black pepper

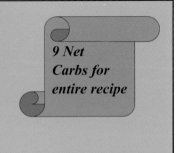

9 Net Carbs for entire recipe

1. Place the basil, nuts, and garlic into a food processor. Process a few times with the pulse button to sufficiently chop the ingredients into small pieces.

2. While the food processor is on, slowly add the olive oil in a continuous stream. Stop occasionally to scrape down the sides with a rubber spatula.

3. Add the cheese and pulse again until fully blended. Add the salt and freshly ground black pepper to taste.

TIP—Make this recipe in large quantities and freeze in a plastic ice cube tray. When you need fresh pesto for a recipe, simply pop out a cube or two and thaw in the microwave.

Zucchini Alfredo

Ingredients
1 tablespoon olive oil
1 cup julienned zucchini (3 net carbs)
¼ cup Rich and Creamy Alfredo Sauce, recipe on
    page 167 (.25 net carb)
¼ cup grated Parmesan or Romano cheese
Salt and freshly ground black pepper

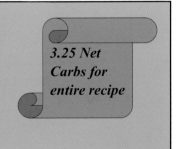

3.25 Net Carbs for entire recipe

Quickly sauté the zucchini in hot olive oil. Add the Alfredo sauce and toss to coat. Sprinkle with the cheese, and grind pepper on top. Salt to taste and serve immediately.

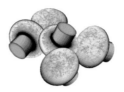

Baked Mushroom Caps with Crabmeat Stuffing

Ingredients
1 cup lump crabmeat
1 large egg (1 net carb)
¼ cup chopped onion (2.5 net carbs)
¼ cup chopped green bell pepper (1.5 net carbs)
¼ cup shredded cheddar cheese
6–8 large mushroom caps (4 net carbs)
Salt and pepper
Hot sauce

9 Net Carbs for entire recipe

1. Preheat the oven to 425 degrees.

2. In a mixing bowl, combine the crabmeat, egg, onion, green pepper, and cheese.

3. Place the mushroom caps on a cookie sheet. Stuff each cap with the crabmeat mixture and bake for 10 to12 minutes, or until the tops of the caps become a nice golden brown color.

4. Salt and pepper to taste, and serve with hot sauce.

TIP—Substitute artichoke hearts for the mushroom caps for Baked Artichoke Hearts with Crabmeat Stuffing.

Cajun Boiled Shrimp

Ingredients

1–2 tablespoons Cajun Land Cajun Seasoning
1 pound large raw, unpeeled shrimp
Butter
1½ cups mixed lettuces (1.5 net carbs)

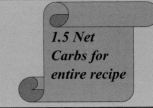

1.5 Net Carbs for entire recipe

Bring 1 quart of water to a boil. Add the Cajun seasoning, then place the shrimp into the water and cook until pink—*do not overcook*. Strain and serve with melted butter and a mixed green salad.

Egg Fu Young

Ingredients

4 large eggs (or 1 cup Egg Beaters) (4 net carbs)
2 cups fresh bean sprouts or 1 can sprouts, well
  drained (8 net carbs)
½ cup chopped scallions (2.5 net carbs)
½ cup diced cooked chicken or ham
1 tablespoon olive oil
Salt and pepper
1 jar Heinz Classic Chicken Gravy, warmed in microwave (12 net carbs)

26.5 Net Carbs for entire recipe

1. Beat the eggs or egg substitute in a mixing bowl until frothy. Add the bean sprouts, scallions, and chicken or ham. Mix well.

2. Heat the olive oil in a nonstick skillet at medium heat. Using a measuring cup, pour ¼ cup of the egg mix into your hot oil. Cook the Egg Fu Young pancakes in a covered skillet, flipping once when the edges become a golden brown. Continue to cook for 2–3 minutes.

3. Salt and pepper to taste and serve immediately, topped with the gravy.

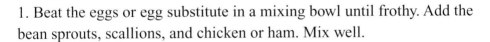

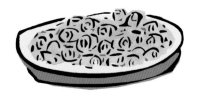

Macafoney and Cheese

Ingredients

1 pound extra-firm tofu, well drained (9 net carbs)
2 cups shredded cheddar cheese
2 large eggs, beaten (2 net carbs)
⅓ cup Rich and Creamy Alfredo Sauce, recipe on
  page 167 (.5 net carb)
¼ cup chopped onion (2.5 net carbs)
Salt and pepper
1 tablespoon melted butter to grease baking dish(es)
½ cup cubed cooked ham (optional)
Grated Parmesan or Romano cheese

14 Net Carbs for entire recipe

1. Preheat the oven to 375 degrees.

2. Cut the tofu into ½-inch cubes. Combine it with the cheese, eggs, Alfredo sauce, and onion, and salt and pepper to taste. If desired, ham can also be added.

3. Pour the mixture into a well-greased, shallow casserole dish, individual baking dishes, or a pie plate. Bake for 30–45 minutes until golden brown and slightly crunchy on top.

4. Sprinkle grated Parmesan or Romano cheese on top prior to serving.

TIP—Freeze uncooked inside individual baking dishes for a fast, easy meal.

Video-supported recipe! Go to this Web site to watch me make it for you: **www.FATtoSKINNY.com/recipes.htm.**

Blackened Fish with Pico de Gallo

This recipe creates smoke, so I suggest you cook it outside on the grill using an oven-safe skillet. I use my cast iron skillets whenever I blacken any food. For blackening seasoning, I like Chef Paul Prudhomme's Magic Seasoning Blends, available in most grocery stores.

Ingredients
¼ cup chopped ripe tomato (1.5 net carbs)
¼ cup chopped onion (2.5 net carbs)
2 tablespoons chopped fresh cilantro (1.5 net carbs)
2 tablespoons chopped fresh parsley (1.5 net carbs)
A squeeze of lemon or lime juice (about a teaspoon)
Salt and pepper
1 6-ounce white fish filet (such as grouper, cod, or haddock), 1-inch thick
2 tablespoons blackening seasoning
2 tablespoons butter

7 Net Carbs for entire recipe

1. For the pico de gallo, combine the tomato, onion, cilantro, parsley, lemon or lime juice, and salt and pepper to taste in a mixing bowl. Set aside.

2. Now let's cook the fish. Heat the grill up to high heat with the skillet on the grill. Generously coat both sides of the fish filet with a good fish-blackening seasoning.

3. When the skillet is very hot, drop in the butter. It will instantly start to sizzle as it melts. Stir it around until the butter starts to smoke, then drop in the fish (be careful of splattering butter).

4. Close the grill lid and cook the fish for 3 to 4 minutes. The cooked side of the fish should be fairly dark. Flip, and cook the second side until the fish starts to split on top. Remove the fish from the skillet.

5. Serve immediately, generously topped with the pico de gallo (use a slotted spoon to avoid too much liquid transferring to the plate).

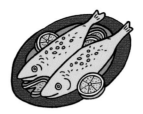

Baked Trout with Zucchini and Bell Pepper

Ingredients
2 teaspoons butter
1 large boneless trout filet
Salt and pepper
¼ cup sliced onion (2.5 net carbs)
2 teaspoons olive oil
½ cup chopped zucchini (1.5 net carbs)
½ cup chopped green bell pepper (3 net carbs)

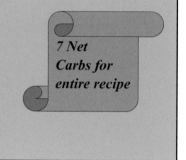

7 Net Carbs for entire recipe

1. Preheat the oven to 375 degrees with a rack in the middle. Line a cookie sheet with foil and grease it with butter.

2. Check the filet for any missed bones and use tweezers to remove any you find. Place the trout filet, skin side down, on the cookie sheet. Salt and pepper the fish to taste and top with the onion slices.

3. Place the fish in the oven and set the timer for 30 minutes.

4. Meanwhile, heat the olive oil in a skillet over medium-high heat. Stir-fry the zucchini and green pepper until they are soft or as you like them. Salt and pepper the veggies to taste.

5. When the fish is flakey, it's done. Remove the fish from the oven and slip a metal spatula between the skin and the flesh. Wiggle the spatula through the fish, separating it from the skin. Serve the fish and vegetables immediately, topped with a pat of butter.

TIP—Don't be afraid of bones. If you can't get a boned filet, proceed with the recipe as described. When the fish is done, simply loosen one end of the skeleton with a fork and gently pull out the entire skeleton. It's much easier to remove the skeleton of a trout after it's cooked.

Chicken Enchilada with Sour Cream and Guacamole

Serves 2

I have found most store-bought brands of enchilada sauce are 3 net carbs per ¼ cup. Check the labels and buy the lowest-carb sauce available in your market. Serve these enchiladas with a green salad.

Ingredients
1 cup chopped cooked chicken
½ cup low-sugar enchilada sauce (6 net carbs)
1 cup shredded cheddar cheese
¼ cup finely chopped onion (2.5 net carbs)
Salt and pepper
2 La Tortilla Factory tortillas (6 net carbs)
¼ cup sour cream (2.5 net carbs)
¼ cup guacamole, recipe follows (2 net carbs)
1 small ripe tomato, chopped, for garnish (3 net carbs)
Small pieces purple cabbage, for garnish

22 Net Carbs for entire recipe

1. Preheat the oven to 375 degrees.

2. Combine the chicken, half the enchilada sauce, ½ cup of the cheese, and the onion, and salt and pepper to taste. Mix well.

3. Spread 1 tablespoon of the enchilada sauce into each of two baking dishes.

4. Divide the chicken mixture into two portions and place each in the center of one of the tortillas. Roll up the tortillas and place, seam side down, in the baking dishes. Spread 1 tablespoon of the sauce over each enchilada and sprinkle ¼ cup of the cheese over the top of each.

5. Bake for 20 to 25 minutes, or until the edges of the tortillas are crisp and the cheese is melted.

6. Remove the enchiladas from the oven and drop a generous dollop of sour cream and guacamole on top of each. Garnish with the tomato and a piece of purple cabbage and serve.

TIP—Freeze uncooked inside individual baking dishes for a fast, easy meal.

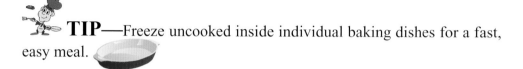

Guacamole

A good ripe avocado for guacamole will be melon-soft when squeezed.

Ingredients
1 ripe Florida avocado (4 net carbs)
¼ cup minced red onion (2.5 net carbs)
1 tablespoon chopped fresh cilantro (1 net carb)
½ tablespoon of fresh lime or lemon juice (.5 net carb)
¼ teaspoon coarse salt
Freshly ground black pepper
1 minced Serrano chile, stems and seeds removed
¼ cup chopped ripe plum tomato, optional (1.5 net carbs)

8 Net Carbs for entire recipe without tomato

1. Cutting an avocado is easy if you know how. Place the avocado on the cutting board. Using a sharp knife, cut the fruit from the top to the bottom. You'll notice the knife is stopped in the center. That's because a big seed is in the way. Turn the avocado over and repeat the same cut, top to bottom, allowing the knife to be stopped by the seed. Make sure you've cut all the way through the fruit above and below the seed. Now the only thing keeping the two halves together is the seed. Take the avocado in hand, one side with one hand, the other side with your other hand. Twist the fruit halves in

opposite directions until they separate. You'll notice one half still has the seed in place. Simply scoop it out with a spoon.

2. Scoop out all the fruit and place it into a mixing bowl. Mash the fruit with a fork until fairly smooth. Add the onion, cilantro, lime or lemon juice, salt, and a few grinds of pepper and mix well.

3. Slowly add the minced chile until the desired heat is achieved. If desired, mix in the chopped plum tomato just prior to serving.

TIP—Guacamole does not keep well. It oxidizes and browns on top. To avoid this, spray a little lemon or lime juice on top and cover with plastic wrap until ready to serve. Only make as much as you'll use in one recipe.

Dungeness Crab

Oh, how I love Dungeness crab! Every time I eat one it brings me back to the San Francisco wharf: fond memories of sitting at the wharf, eating one of these wonderful crabs and, of course, that famous San Fran sourdough bread! Well, the bread is history for me now, but I'm proud to announce that Dungeness is still on the menu.

Ingredients
1 Dungeness crab
2–3 tablespoons butter
1 cup green salad (2 net carbs)

2 Net Carbs for entire recipe

1. When you buy one of these crabs from your local market, they are already cooked. All you need to do is place a thawed crab in a steamer *above* the water level and heat it up for about 6 minutes. Don't immerse the crab in water or you'll wash out the natural salts in the flesh and the crab will taste bland.

2. Melt some butter to dip the crab into, make a nice salad, and dig in!

Eggplant Parmesan with Fresh Spinach

When you buy eggplant, look for a fruit that has a fairly consistent purple color all around. Brown spots on the outside are the first sign that the eggplant is browning on the inside. I have found that store-bought pasta sauce carb counts vary widely. Be diligent and read the labels. The lowest I've found in most stores is 4 net carbs per ½ cup.

Ingredients
1 small eggplant (6 net carbs)
¼ cup olive oil
Salt and pepper
1 large egg (1 net carb)
2 tablespoons cream
1 cup Fry Coating (recipe on page 251)
½ cup low-sugar pasta sauce (4 net carbs)
½ cup shredded mozzarella cheese
1 cup fresh spinach, packed (1 net carb)
1 teaspoon balsamic vinegar (1 net carb)

13 Net Carbs for entire recipe

1. Preheat the oven to 350 degrees.

2. Peel the eggplant and slice it into rounds ¼- to ½-inch thick.

3. Heat the olive oil in a nonstick skillet over medium heat. Olive oil has a low smoke point and we don't want to burn the oil.

4. Salt and pepper the eggplant rounds. Beat the egg with the cream in a medium bowl. Dredge the eggplant rounds in the egg wash, then in the Fry Coating.

5. Once you have three rounds ready, gently drop them into the hot oil and continue dredging the remainder.

6. Flip the sizzling rounds over when the bottoms show a nice brown circle around the outside edge. Continue to cook the rounds until both sides are golden brown.

7. Remove the rounds and place them on a paper towel to drain while the others cook.

8. Spread a light coating of pasta sauce on a cookie sheet and layer 4 fried eggplant rounds, overlapping each other a bit. Spread a little more pasta sauce across the top of the rounds and top with a sprinkling of mozzarella.

9. Place the cookie sheet into the hot oven for 10 to 15 minutes or until the cheese is melted and bubbly. Using a large spatula, transfer the eggplant onto a dinner plate.

10. In a separate bowl, toss the fresh spinach with a sprinkling of olive oil, the balsamic vinegar, and a pinch of salt and pepper. Arrange the spinach around the outside of the plate, surrounding the eggplant, and serve.

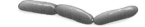 **TIP**—Freeze uncooked inside individual baking dishes for a fast, easy meal.

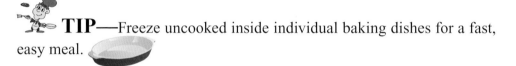

Italian Sausage and Onions

Ingredients
1 tablespoon olive oil
5 Italian sausages, hot, sweet, or mild (5 net carbs)
½ cup low-sugar pasta sauce (4 net carbs)
½ cup sliced onion (5 net carbs)
1 tablespoon chopped fresh parsley (1 net carb)
Salt and pepper

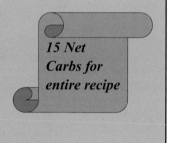

15 Net Carbs for entire recipe

1. Heat the olive oil in a skillet over medium heat and cook the sausages in the oil. Poke a fork into a couple of the sausages to release some of the juices into the pan.

2. When they are brown on all sides, remove the sausages and sauté the onion until golden brown.

3. Place the sausages back into the pan with the onion. Pour in the pasta sauce and stir. Cover and reduce the heat to medium-low. Simmer for 10

minutes. Uncover and sprinkle parsley over the top, add salt and pepper to taste, stir, and serve.

Wilted Zucchini with Grated Romano

Ah, pasta—I love anything that even resembles pasta. ☺ Zucchini makes a wonderful replacement for pasta and is much more flavorful. This dish is perfect for a light lunch or as a side dish for dinner.

Ingredients
1 tablespoon butter
1 teaspoon olive oil
1½ cups julienned zucchini (4.5 net carbs)
Freshly ground black pepper
½ teaspoon coarse salt
¼ cup grated Romano cheese
1 tablespoon fresh basil, finely chopped (1 net carb)

5.5 Net Carbs for entire recipe

1. Heat the butter and olive oil in a skillet over medium heat. Watch it—you don't want to burn the butter.

2. Toss in the zucchini and quickly stir-fry for 2 to 3 minutes, then remove from the heat and grind in some pepper along with the salt.

3. Mix in the cheese and basil and serve.

TIP—I use a tabletop V-slicer, also known as a kitchen mandoline, to prepare my zucchini. It quickly makes evenly sized pieces. They are readily available, fairly inexpensive, and a great tool in the kitchen.

Shrimp Lo Mein with Sweet Red Peppers and Scallions

Buy Miracle Noodles from: www.miraclenoodle.com. They are a wonderful product replacing traditional pasta and they are completely sugar-free.

Ingredients
1 package Miracle Noodles Angel Hair Pasta
1 tablespoon butter
½ pound medium shrimp, peeled and deveined
½ cup julienned red bell pepper (3 net carbs)
1 tablespoon sugar-free teriyaki sauce
1 tablespoon soy sauce (1 net carb)
2 scallions, chopped (.5 net carbs)
Salt and pepper

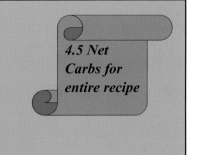

4.5 Net Carbs for entire recipe

1. Start by opening the package of noodles. They are already cooked, so simply drop them in a strainer and rinse well.

2. While the noodles are draining, melt the butter over medium-high heat in a nonstick skillet.

3. Peel the shrimp. Quickly sauté the shrimp and bell pepper in the melted butter until the shrimp turn reddish in color. Remove the shrimp and bell pepper and set aside in a bowl, making sure to reserve the liquids in the pan.

4. Place the teriyaki sauce, soy sauce, and Miracle Noodles in the pan and cook for 2 to 3 minutes, stirring well to completely coat the noodles with the sauce.

5. Remove the noodles from the pan and place in the bowl with the shrimp and peppers, once again reserving the liquid.

6. Increase the temperature to high and bring the liquid in the pan to a boil. Reduce the liquid to a syrupy consistency and remove from heat.

7. Toss all the ingredients back into the pan, including the chopped scallion, and mix well.

8. Salt and pepper to taste and serve with a green side salad.

The Savory Salads

I love all the savory salads as toppings on a green salad, stuffed into a nice big fat tomato, or simply eaten as a wrap in a romaine lettuce leaf or a low-carb tortilla. The basics for each of the following are almost the same; the biggest difference is the main ingredient.

Savory Salad Base

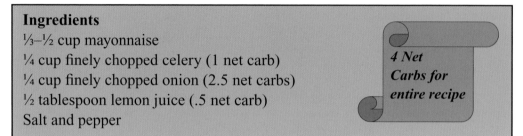

Ingredients
⅓–½ cup mayonnaise
¼ cup finely chopped celery (1 net carb)
¼ cup finely chopped onion (2.5 net carbs)
½ tablespoon lemon juice (.5 net carb)
Salt and pepper

4 Net Carbs for entire recipe

Combine all the ingredients and mix well. Follow one of the variations below.

Egg Salad

Omit the lemon juice. Add 2 or 3 hard-cooked eggs, chopped to your size preference. Add 1 net carb per egg.

Chicken Salad

Add ½ to ¾ cup chopped cooked chicken and ½ teaspoon chopped fresh thyme.

Tuna Salad

Add ½ to ¾ cup canned tuna. Optionally, add 1 teaspoon finely chopped jalapeño pepper if you wish to spice it up. Make sure to wash your hands well after chopping the pepper. Also try adding 1 tablespoon chopped black olives.

Ham Salad

Add ½ to ¾ cup chopped cooked ham. I like to use the ham from a baked ham dinner. Optionally, add a pinch of ground cloves and a pinch of ground nutmeg for that "surprise" flavor.

Salmon Salad

Add ½ to ¾ cup chopped cooked salmon. When I have salmon for dinner I always pan-fry an additional filet for salmon salad. Optionally, add 1 to 2 teaspoons capers. Change the chopped white onion to chopped red onion for a stronger flavor.

Turkey and Red Cabbage Salad

Add ½ to ¾ cup chopped cooked turkey, ½ teaspoon chopped fresh thyme, and ½ cup roughly chopped purple cabbage.

WRAPS AND MELTS

Savory Salad Wraps and Melts

Wrap any of the savory salads in fresh romaine lettuce leaves for a wonderful cold lunch, or turn your lunch into a hot meal by changing the wrap to a low-carb tortilla: scoop on any of the savory salads, top it with a good serving of shredded cheddar cheese, and microwave for 30 seconds to melt the cheese.

Chicken Parmesan Wrap

Ingredients
1 tablespoon olive oil
1 boneless, skinless chicken breast
3 tablespoons low-sugar pasta sauce (1 net carb)
¼ cup shredded mozzarella cheese
2 large romaine lettuce leaves (1 net carb) or 1 La
   Tortilla Factory tortilla (3 net carbs)
Parmesan cheese
Salt and pepper

2 Net Carbs for entire recipe with lettuce

1. Heat the oil in a nonstick skillet over medium-high heat.

2. While the oil is heating, place the chicken breast in a gallon-size zippered plastic bag. Zip the bag most of the way shut, leaving a small open-

ing. Place the bag on a cutting board and pound the breast with a rolling pin or wine bottle to a ¼-inch thickness.

3. Salt and pepper both sides of the chicken and fry for 3 to 4 minutes per side, making sure all pinkness has disappeared from the poultry. Spoon the pasta sauce over the breast and cover with cheese. Place a lid on the skillet and reduce the heat to low. Continue to heat 2 to 3 minutes more, or until the cheese is melted.

4. Transfer the chicken to a cutting board and slice it in half to make two nice wraps on romaine leaves. Sprinkle a generous amount of Parmesan cheese on top and enjoy!

Philly Cheese Steak Wrap

I like London broil for this wrap, but you can use the steak of your choice.

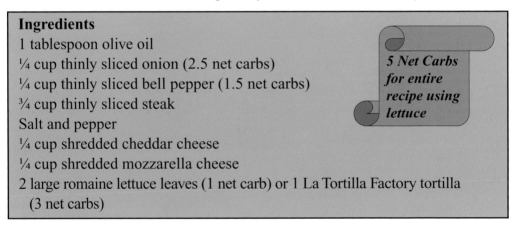

Ingredients
1 tablespoon olive oil
¼ cup thinly sliced onion (2.5 net carbs)
¼ cup thinly sliced bell pepper (1.5 net carbs)
¾ cup thinly sliced steak
Salt and pepper
¼ cup shredded cheddar cheese
¼ cup shredded mozzarella cheese
2 large romaine lettuce leaves (1 net carb) or 1 La Tortilla Factory tortilla
  (3 net carbs)

5 Net Carbs for entire recipe using lettuce

1. Heat the oil in a nonstick skillet over medium-high heat. Sauté the onion and pepper until soft. Add the steak and stir-fry until done to your preference. Salt and pepper the meat and veggies and throw in the cheese. Cover the pan and remove from the heat.

2. Spread out the lettuce or tortilla and uncover the pan. Quickly stir the mixture until the cheese is well incorporated with the veggies and meat. Scoop the mixture into the wrap and serve with a dill pickle and EatSmart Soy Crisps.

TIP—When slicing the steak, slice individual portions and freeze in a freezer bag for a quick and easy lunch.

Pepper and Egg Wrap

You can use either red or green bell pepper in this dish. Red pepper will make the dish a bit sweeter, the green a bit tangy.

Ingredients

½ tablespoon butter

¼ cup julienned red or green bell pepper (1.5 net carbs)

2 large eggs (2 net carbs)

2 tablespoons shredded smoked Gouda cheese

1 large romaine lettuce leaf (.5 net carb) or 1 La
   Tortilla Factory tortilla (3 net carbs)

2 tablespoons low-sugar salsa, room temperature (1 net carb)

Salt and pepper

5 Net Carbs for entire recipe using lettuce

1. Melt the butter in a nonstick skillet over medium heat. When the butter is melted, toss in the bell pepper. Stir-fry the peppers for 2 to 3 minutes or until soft.

2. Whisk the eggs well and pour them into the skillet on top of the peppers. Cover and reduce the heat to medium-low. Check the eggs in 2 to 3 minutes. Using a spatula, gently lift up one side of the omelet an inch or so, then tilt the pan so raw egg flows under the cooked egg. Repeat on the other side.

3. Sprinkle the cheese over the top of the omelet and cover. Wait 30 seconds, then turn off the heat.

4. Open the lid and lay the lettuce or tortilla over the top of the omelet. Place a serving plate face-down on top of the pan and using two hands—one on top of the plate, holding it in place, and one on the skillet handle—invert the pan so the omelet falls out of the pan onto the plate. Wow, that was fun! ☺

5. Now spread the salsa on the omelet, salt and pepper to taste, and serve.

Roast Beef Melt

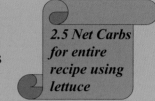

Ingredients
1 large romaine lettuce leaf (.5 net carb) or 1 La
   Tortilla Factory tortilla (3 net carbs)
1 tablespoon horseradish mayonnaise, recipe follows
½ cup shredded lettuce (.5 net carb)
2–3 thin tomato slices (1 net carb)
2–3 thin garlic dill pickle slices (.5 net carb)
Salt and pepper
¾ cup thinly sliced roast beef
2 slices or ¼ cup shredded horseradish cheese

2.5 Net Carbs for entire recipe using lettuce

1. Place the romaine leaf onto your serving plate and evenly spread the horseradish mayo onto the lettuce. Next, stack the veggies on top—shredded lettuce first, then tomato, then pickles. Salt and pepper the veggies. Careful, you'll be seasoning the meat as well.

2. Place a piece of foil on a cookie sheet and stack the meat in the center of the foil. Season the meat with a bit of salt and pepper. Cover the meat with the cheese and place under the broiler until the cheese is melted and bubbly.

3. Using a spatula, scoop up the meat from the foil and place it on top of the veggies. Fold over the leaf and enjoy.

Horseradish Mayonnaise—Mix 2 tablespoons mayonnaise, 1 teaspoon prepared horseradish, a dash of salt and pepper, and ½ teaspoon fresh chopped parsley.

TIP—To make this using a tortilla, place the tortilla on a cookie sheet. Evenly spread the horseradish mayo on the tortilla. Next, stack the veggies on top of the tortilla—shredded lettuce first, then tomato, then pickles. Salt and pepper the veggies. Careful, you'll be seasoning the meat as well. Now cover the veggies with the beef and season again. Top it all off with the cheese. Place the wrap under a hot broiler just long enough to make the cheese bubbly. Plate and serve.

Lamb Melt

Ingredients
1 La Tortilla Factory tortilla (3 net carbs)
1 teaspoon mayonnaise
1 teaspoon Dijon mustard (.5 carbs)
¾ cup thinly sliced cooked lamb
¼ cup thinly sliced onion (2.5 net carbs)
Salt and pepper
¼ cup crumbled feta cheese

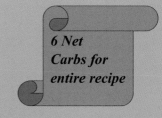

6 Net Carbs for entire recipe

1. Place the tortilla on a cookie sheet. Mix the mayonnaise and mustard together. Evenly spread the mix on the tortilla.

2. Next, layer on the sliced lamb and the onion. Salt and pepper to taste and top with the feta cheese.

3. Place the wrap under a hot broiler just long enough to make the cheese bubbly. Serve immediately.

DINNER

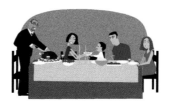

Grilled Peppers and Steak with Rosemary-infused Olive Oil

There are several different types of steaks out there to choose from, so which one do you choose? In the back of this book you'll find the answers. I've outlined suggestions for you, well . . . for my wife and for you.

For this recipe I've chosen Delmonico. These steaks are tender, carry a medium marbling, and hold up well against high heat on the grill, in comparison to, say, a rib eye. In my neck of the woods, a rib eye is a steak cut from the roast prime rib. Rib eye steaks usually carry a high amount of fat and flare-ups become a major problem on a grill. They are best cooked at a lower heat or on a flameless grill surface. Another good choice for this recipe would be porterhouse or T-bone.

I personally like my meat rare. The truth of it is, the rarer your meat is cooked, the more tender it will be.

Ingredients
½ red bell pepper (1.5 net carbs)
½ yellow bell pepper (1.5 net carbs)
6-ounce Delmonico steak, or another steak of your choice
1 tablespoon Rosemary-infused Olive Oil, recipe follows
Coarse salt and freshly ground black pepper

3 Net Carbs for entire recipe

1. Start by heating up the grill. A good hot grill prevents sticking and gives you those really great grill marks.

2. While the grill is heating up, squash the peppers flat on the cutting

board, using the palm of your hand. Baste the steaks and peppers with rosemary oil and generously salt and pepper.

3. Place the steak and peppers on the hot grill and cook to desired doneness (see steak grilling chart on page 300). I recommend NOT closing the grill cover when cooking thinner steaks.

4. Serve with Caulimash, recipe follows.

Rosemary-infused Olive Oil—Making infused oils is very easy. To make this oil, simply buy a bottle of olive oil, pop off the top, and take out a few tablespoons of oil. Slide a sprig of fresh rosemary into the bottle, making certain to cover the entire sprig with oil to prevent mold. If you need to top off the bottle, use the oil that you drained at the beginning. Place the cap back on the oil and place it in the pantry. In a week or two the oil will be ready. The longer it marinates, the stronger the rosemary flavor will be. Remove the cap and take out the rosemary sprig and discard. The oil is now ready for use in your favorite recipes or on your next salad.

Caulimash

Benecol contains plant sterols, a natural cholesterol reducer. Although it's lousy to use for cooking, it works great as an additive or spread.

Ingredients
1 head cauliflower (1.5 net carbs per ½ cup)
2 tablespoons mayonnaise
1 tablespoon butter or Benecol spread
Salt and pepper

1.5 Net Carbs per ½ cup serving

1. Steam a head of cauliflower in a couple of inches of water until fork-tender.

2. Drain the cauliflower and place it into a food processor with a chopping blade. Add the mayonnaise, butter or Benecol spread, and salt and pepper to taste.

3. Process until smooth. You now have your "mashed potatoes," or Caulimash.

TIP—To make garlic Caulimash, dice 2 cloves of garlic and add it to the food processor with the cauliflower, mayonnaise, and butter or Benecol. If you want a milder garlic flavor, simply sauté the diced garlic in butter for a few minutes prior to adding it to the food processor. Two cloves of garlic adds 2 carbs to the recipe's net carb count.

To make cheesy Caulimash, add ½ cup shredded cheddar cheese to the food processor before blending. Cheese adds no additional carbs.

To make Mexican Caulimash, add ½ teaspoon each of cayenne pepper, chili powder, and ground cumin before blending. The spices add no additional carbs.

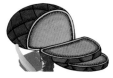

Baked Ham with Broccoli and Caulimash

There are a variety of hams on the market in your grocer's meat case. The average low-SUGAR ham ranges from 0 to 4 carbs per serving. The carb count will depend on whether they use sugar in the curing process or offer a glaze on the ham. Find the lowest carb count ham for your dinner. If you find one that's 0 carbs, make a note of the brand for future meals. The shank portion of the ham is usually less money; however, it contains a larger bone. I like the butt portion myself.

Ingredients
½ ham, shank or butt portion
1 tablespoon butter or Benecol spread
Salt and pepper
1 head broccoli (2 net carbs per ½ cup)
0-carb mustard

3.5 Net Carbs per serving with Caulimash

1. Bake the ham following the package instructions.

2. Prepare your Caulimash as directed on page 197.

3. Using the same pot in which you cooked your cauliflower, bring an inch of salted water to a boil.

4. Cut an inch off the bottom of the broccoli and, using a sharp knife, peel the stem and quarter the broccoli. Place the broccoli into the pot, cover, and cook to your desired tenderness. (I like my broccoli crisp so I only steam it for about 5 minutes. If you like yours a bit softer increase the steaming time to as long as 10 minutes.) Drain well and melt the remaining tablespoon of butter over the top.

5. Slice the ham with a sharp knife.

6. Serve the ham, Caulimash, and broccoli with extra butter and the 0-carb mustard of your choice.

TIP—Cut a couple of thick slices of ham into cubes. Stick a green olive on a toothpick and stab the ham cube. Repeat until you run out of ham and olives. Store in the fridge for a snack tray.

Chicken Cordon Bleu with Sesame Stir-Fry

Use leftovers from a baked ham dinner for the ham.

Ingredients
1 slice Swiss cheese
1 thin slice ham
1 boneless, skinless chicken breast
1 tablespoon olive oil
¼ cup julienned red bell pepper (1.5 net carbs)
¼ cup julienned yellow bell pepper (1.5 net carbs)
¼ cup julienned zucchini (.75 net carbs)
1 tablespoon sesame seeds

3.75 Net Carbs for entire recipe

Salt and pepper
½ tablespoon butter

1. Preheat the oven to 375 degrees.

2. Place the slice of cheese on top of the slice of ham and roll it up. Using a sharp knife, cut a pocket inside the chicken breast. Stuff the rolled ham and cheese into the pocket and close with a wooden toothpick.

3. Bake for 35 minutes, then remove it from the oven, cover it with foil, and set aside.

4. Heat the olive oil in a skillet over medium-high heat. Toss in the bell peppers, zucchini, and sesame seeds. Salt and pepper the veggies and quickly stir-fry. Remove while still crisp and plate, topping with the butter.

5. Remove the chicken from the baking dish and, with a sharp knife, slice into ½-inch slices. Salt and pepper to taste and serve.

TIP—Make a couple of extra chicken cordon bleus and place them in the fridge to cool. In the morning, slice the breasts into pinwheels and place them on a tray in the fridge for snacks. Freeze uncooked inside individual baking dishes for a fast, easy dinner.

Video-supported recipe! Go to this Web site to watch me make it for you: **www.FATtoSKINNY.com/recipes.htm**.

Corned Beef and Cabbage Boil

Buy a fresh corned beef from the grocer for this hearty dinner.

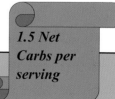

1.5 Net Carbs per serving

Ingredients
1 corned beef

1 head green cabbage, cut into wedges (1.5 net carbs per ½ cup)
0 carb mustard

1. Boil the corned beef following the package instructions.

2. When the beef is fork-tender, add wedges of cabbage to the water. Cook the cabbage until it reaches your desired tenderness.

3. Serve with your favorite 0-carb mustard.

TIP—Put leftover corned beef into a food processor and chop for breakfast corned beef hash (see page 142).

Cajun Seafood Boil

Serves 4

Use any white fish filets of your choice; I prefer grouper or cod. You will need cheesecloth and twist ties to prepare the fish.

Ingredients
2–3 tablespoons Cajun Land Cajun Seasoning
4 white fish filets
1 small head green cabbage, cut into wedges (1.5 net carbs per ½ cup)
2 onions, cut in half (5 net carbs per ½ cup)
2 cups green beans (3 net carbs per ½ cup)
1 pound raw, unpeeled shrimp, fresh or thawed if frozen
4 tablespoons salted butter, melted

9.5 Net Carbs per serving

1. Bring 2 quarts of water to a boil in a large pot. Add the Cajun seasoning.

2. Enclose each filet in a cheesecloth wrap pulled into a sack and tied with a twist tie. Drop the fish bags into the water along with the cabbage

wedges, onions, and green beans. Boil for about 10 minutes, or until cabbage is fork-tender but not mushy.

3. Add the shrimp. Boil another 2 to 3 minutes, or until the shrimp is pink.

4. Melt the butter in the microwave in a covered microwave-safe dish.

5. Set up plates with a small dish of melted butter for dipping, a serving of veggies, shrimp, and a fish bag in the center and serve.

TIP—Cook extra fish and shrimp to chop the next day for Cajun Seafood Salad (see page 174).

Macafoney and Cheese Primavera

Ingredients
1 pound extra-firm tofu (9 net carbs; 2 net carbs per ½ cup)
2 cups shredded cheddar cheese
½ cup Rich and Creamy Alfredo Sauce, recipe on page 167 (5 net carb)

5 Net Carbs per 1 cup serving

2 large eggs, beaten (2 net carbs)
¼ cup chopped onion (2.5 net carbs)
¼ cup chopped red bell pepper (1.5 net carbs)
¼ cup chopped yellow bell pepper (1.5 net carbs)
¼ cup chopped mushrooms (1 net carb)
2 teaspoons butter to grease casserole dish(es)
Salt and pepper
2 tablespoons grated Parmesan or Romano cheese
Fresh basil leaves, for garnish

1. Preheat the oven to 375 degrees.

2. Drain the tofu well and cut it into ½-inch cubes. In a mixing bowl, combine the tofu with the cheddar cheese, Alfredo sauce, eggs, onion, bell peppers, mushrooms, and salt and pepper to taste.

3. Pour the mixture into a well-greased, shallow casserole dish, individual casseroles, or a pie plate.

4. Bake for 30 to 45 minutes, until golden brown and slightly crunchy on top. Sprinkle the Parmesan or Romano cheese on top, garnish with a basil leaf, and serve.

TIP—Freeze uncooked portion inside individual baking dishes for a fast, easy meal. Add chopped ham or leftover chopped chicken for a hearty variation.

Video-supported recipe! Go to this Web site to watch me make it for you: **www.FATtoSKINNY.com/recipes.htm**.

Italian Stuffed Chicken Breast with Romano Green Beans

Serves 4

Use your favorite low-SUGAR tomato-based pasta sauce for this dinner.

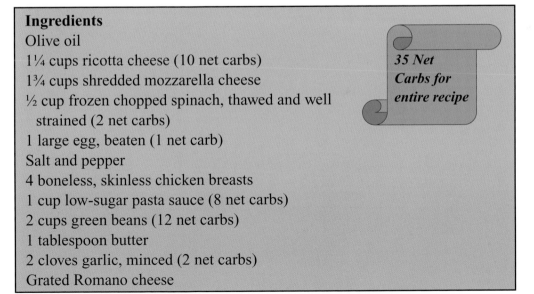

Ingredients
Olive oil
1¼ cups ricotta cheese (10 net carbs)
1¾ cups shredded mozzarella cheese
½ cup frozen chopped spinach, thawed and well
   strained (2 net carbs)
1 large egg, beaten (1 net carb)
Salt and pepper
4 boneless, skinless chicken breasts
1 cup low-sugar pasta sauce (8 net carbs)
2 cups green beans (12 net carbs)
1 tablespoon butter
2 cloves garlic, minced (2 net carbs)
Grated Romano cheese

35 Net Carbs for entire recipe

1. Preheat the oven to 350-degrees. Grease 4 individual baking dishes with olive oil.

2. In a mixing bowl, combine the ricotta cheese, ¾ cup of mozzarella cheese, spinach, egg, and salt and pepper to taste. Mix well and transfer to a gallon-size zippered plastic bag.

3. Using a sharp knife, cut a pocket inside each chicken breast. Cut a SMALL corner off the plastic bag and pipe the filling into the pockets, about ⅓ cup for each breast. Close with a wooden toothpick.

4. Place the breasts into the baking dishes. Ladle ¼ cup of the pasta sauce over each breast, sprinkle ¼ cup of the mozzarella cheese on top of each, and bake for 30 minutes. Cheese should be melted and lightly browned around the edges.

5. Steam the green beans for 5 minutes. (They should still be crisp when removed from the steamer.) Place them into a skillet with the butter, 2 tablespoons olive oil, and garlic. Sauté for 3 to 5 minutes, or until the beans are softened to your liking.

6. Serve the chicken and green beans with a generous amount of Romano cheese on top.

TIP—Make a couple of extra chicken breasts and refrigerate. In the morning, slice the breasts into pinwheels and keep on a tray in fridge for snacks. Freeze uncooked portions inside individual baking dishes for a fast, easy dinner.

Bacon-Wrapped Filet Mignon with Garlic Caulimash and Broccoli

Ingredients
2 6-ounce filet mignon steaks
2 slices turkey bacon

1 tablespoon olive oil
1 tablespoon Montreal steak seasoning
1 small head broccoli (2 net carbs per ½ cup)
1 tablespoon salted butter, melted

9.5 Net Carbs per serving including Caulimash

1. Prepare the Caulimash as directed on page 197, using the garlic method described in the Tip section. Set aside and reheat in a microwave-safe container before serving.

2. Place a saucepan with an inch of water in the bottom on the stovetop over high heat.

3. Trim off the bottom inch from the broccoli stem. Next, stand the broccoli on its stem and, using a sharp knife, pare off the skin of the stem in steady downward strokes. Lay the broccoli on its side and cut it in half lengthwise.

4. Place the broccoli in the boiling water and cover, cooking for 3 minutes. Remove the broccoli and drain, leaving it in the colander until serving time. When serving, drizzle hot melted butter over the top of each broccoli serving.

5. Heat the grill on high heat.

6. While the grill is heating, wrap a piece of turkey bacon around each filet and hold in place with toothpicks. I prefer turkey bacon because it's fully cooked already. If you eat your meat rare or medium-rare, the cooking time is short and pork bacon doesn't have time to cook through.

7. Brush the steaks and bacon with olive oil, then coat with Montreal steak seasoning. Place on the hot grill and close the lid. The filet and the turkey bacon are low in fat, so flare-ups should not be a problem.

8. After 3 or 4 minutes of cooking on very high heat, lift the steaks with tongs and take a look. The filets should now have attractive grill marks and the first ¼ inch of meat should be browned nicely. If not, place the steaks back on the grill and check again in a couple of minutes.

9. When ready, flip the steaks once and finish the cooking process over high heat with an open lid. Cook to desired doneness and serve with steamed broccoli and Caulimash.

Shrimp Scampi on Spaghetti Squash

Ingredients
1 medium spaghetti squash (6 net carbs per ¾ cup)
2 tablespoons olive oil
1 tablespoon butter
3 cloves garlic, minced (3 net carbs)
1½ pounds large raw shrimp, peeled and deveined
Salt and pepper
Grated Parmesan or Romano cheese
1½ cups fresh spinach (1.5 net carbs)
2 tablespoons feta cheese (1 net carb)
5 green olives, chopped (2.5 net carbs)

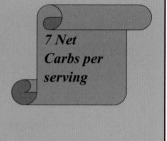

7 Net Carbs per serving

1. Punch 10 or 12 steam vent holes about 2 inches deep into the spaghetti squash with a sharp knife. Place the spaghetti squash in the microwave and cook on high for about 20 minutes. To test doneness, gently squeeze with a gloved hand (it will be hot). If the squash gives, then it's done. If not, cook longer, checking at 5-minute intervals until it is soft enough to give when squeezed.

2. When the squash is done, place it on a cutting board and allow to cool for 10 minutes. Cut it in half lengthwise, then let stand to cool.

3. Heat the olive oil and butter in skillet over medium heat. Sauté the garlic in the skillet until it is lightly browned. Add the shrimp to the skillet and sauté until the shrimp become pink. Remove the skillet from the heat.

4. With a fork, remove the seeds from the squash and discard. Now, using the fork, start pulling the squash meat out onto a plate. Notice that the meat looks like strands of angel hair pasta, which is why it's called spaghetti squash. Salt and pepper the squash to taste and toss with Romano or Parmesan cheese.

5. Once the squash is "dressed," transfer ¾-cup portions to dinner plates and smother with the shrimp mixture.

6. Serve with a spinach salad topped with feta cheese and olives.

Roast Turkey with Caulimash and Baked Asparagus

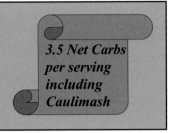

Ingredients
1 small whole turkey, about 12 pounds
15 asparagus spears (2 net carbs per 5 spears)
1 tablespoon olive oil
Grated Parmesan or Romano cheese
Salt and pepper

3.5 Net Carbs per serving including Caulimash

1. Roast the turkey in a roasting pan following the package instructions. (See the roasting chart for poultry on page 310 for roasting times.)

2. Meanwhile, prepare the Caulimash as directed on page 197, using the cheese method described in the Tip section.

3. When the turkey is roasted, remove it from the oven and let it rest while you roast the asparagus.

4. Cut an inch off the bottoms of the asparagus spears and place them in a shallow baking dish. Brush the stalks with olive oil and salt and pepper to taste.

5. Bake at 350 degrees for 20 to 30 minutes, or until fork-tender.

6. Roll the asparagus once in the baking dish to pick up the remaining olive oil and then transfer to a serving plate. Sprinkle Parmesan or Romano cheese on top and season with pepper from a pepper grinder.

7. Serve the turkey with the Caulimash and asparagus.

TIP—Buy a large enough turkey or turkey breast so you have plenty of leftovers for snack trays, lunch meat, and chef's salad toppings.

BBQ Steak and Drumsticks with Grilled Vegetables

Serves 2

Ingredients
1 pound chicken drumsticks
Walden Farms BBQ Sauce
2 4-ounce steaks
1 zucchini (1.5 net carbs per ½ cup)
1 yellow summer squash (1.5 net carbs per ½ cup)
1 red bell pepper (1.5 net carbs per ½ pepper)
1 tablespoon olive oil
Salt and pepper

4.5 Net Carbs per serving

1. Preheat the grill.

2. Cook the chicken drumsticks as directed by the poultry grilling chart on page 312.

3. When the drumsticks are almost done, coat with Walden Farms BBQ Sauce and move them to the outside edges of your grill.

4. Grill your favorite steaks any way you like (avoid any marinades that contain SUGAR or carbs).

5. Slice the zucchini lengthwise and the yellow squash into ½-inch-thick slices. Slice the bell pepper in half, trim, and flatten. Brush all the vegetables with olive oil, salt and pepper each side, and grill until soft, flipping once.

TIP—Slice additional steaks into strips and freeze some of the strips in single servings for Philly Cheese Steak Wraps (see recipe page 192). Skewer the rest onto bamboo skewers, paint with soy sauce, and grill. Place in the fridge along with the leftover chicken drumsticks for snack trays.

Baked Salmon and Fennel in Parchment Paper with Sweet Lemon-Caper Sauce

Serves 2

Ingredients
2 salmon steaks or filets
1 bulb fennel, cut in half (4 net carbs)
6 tablespoons butter
Salt and pepper
1 tablespoon lemon juice (1 net carb)
1 tablespoon capers
1 teaspoon xylitol or stevia
2 cups mixed lettuces (2 net carbs)

9.5 Net Carbs for entire recipe

1. Preheat the oven to 350 degrees.

2. Cut 4 12-inch-square pieces of parchment paper. Place each piece of salmon in the middle of a square. If you're using filets, place them skin side down. Next to the fish, place half a fennel bulb.

3. Melt 2 tablespoons of the butter in the microwave. Paint the fish and fennel with melted butter and season everything with salt and pepper to taste.

4. Loosely place another piece of parchment paper on top of the food and fold the 4 edges together to form a pouch, much like you would do if you were using aluminum foil. The top piece should be an inch or so above the food when the pouch is complete and sealed around all 4 edges. Cut a small slit in the top to allow steam to escape. Place the packages on a cookie sheet and bake for 30 minutes.

5. Melt the remaining 4 tablespoons butter in the microwave. To the melted butter, add the lemon juice, capers, and xylitol or stevia.

6. Serve the packages sealed on dinner plates, allowing diners to open their packages themselves. Spoon the sauce over the fish and fennel when served. Serve with a green salad on the side.

TIP—Cook an extra piece of fish and put it in the fridge to cool. Once cool, remove the skin and place the fish in a food processor with 1 to 2 tablespoons mayonnaise. Process until smooth, mix in finely chopped onion and capers, and salt and pepper for a wonderful salmon spread on GG Bran Crispbread.

Roast Cajun Pork Loin with Creamed Spinach Alfredo and Mushrooms

Cajun Land Cajun Seasoning is available at **www.cajunlandbrand.com**.

Ingredients
2 tablespoons olive oil
2 pounds pork loin
2 tablespoons Cajun Land Cajun Seasoning
1½ cups frozen chopped spinach, thawed and well
   drained (6 net carbs)
½ cup chopped mushrooms (2 net carbs)
½ cup Rich and Creamy Alfredo Sauce, recipe on page 167 (.5 net carb)
1 clove garlic, minced (1 net carb)
¼ cup shredded cheddar cheese
Salt and pepper

9.5 Net Carbs for entire recipe

1. Preheat the oven to 375 degrees.

2. Heat the olive oil in an oven-proof skillet over medium-high heat.

3. Score (in several places and ¼-inch deep) the fat side of the pork loin roast with a sharp knife. Rub the entire roast with Cajun seasoning.

4. Sear all sides of the roast for 2 to 3 minutes in the hot oil. Once seared, place the skillet in the oven and roast for 40 minutes or until a meat thermometer inserted in the loin reads 130 degrees.

5. When the roast reaches 130 degrees, remove it from the oven and let it stand for 15 minutes on the counter.

6. In another skillet, heat up the spinach, mushrooms, Alfredo sauce, and garlic. Continue to cook over medium-low heat until the mushrooms are cooked through. Sprinkle the cheddar cheese on top, then cover and remove from heat.

7. Slice the roast into ¼-inch-thick slices.

8. Ladle a serving of creamed spinach alfredo onto half of a dinner plate and place slices of the pork roast onto the other side of the plate, slightly overlapping the creamed spinach and each previous slice.

TIP—Make a double batch of the spinach for Crepes Florentine filling (page 151).

Grouper Florentine with Baby Greens and Dill Dressing

Serves 2

Makoto Dill Dressing is available at **www.makotodressing.com**.

Ingredients
4 teaspoons butter
1½ cups frozen chopped spinach, thawed and well drained (6 net carbs)
½ cup Rich and Creamy Alfredo Sauce, recipe on page 167 (.5 net carb)
¼ cup roughly chopped onion (2.5 net carbs)
¼ cup cooking sherry
¼ cup shredded cheddar cheese
2 cloves garlic, minced (2 net carbs)
2 6-ounce grouper filets
Salt and pepper

13 Net Carbs for entire recipe

2 cups baby greens (2 net carbs)
Makoto Dill Dressing

1. Preheat the oven to 400 degrees. Butter 2 individual baking dishes with a teaspoon of butter each.

2. Squeeze the spinach to remove excess water and place in a mixing bowl. Add the Alfredo sauce, onion, sherry, cheddar cheese, and garlic, and mix up the "goop." ☺ Split the goop between the baking dishes.

3. Place the grouper into the goop and press down, then flip the filet over and salt and pepper it. Top each filet with a teaspoon of the butter and bake for 25 to 30 minutes, or until the fish is flakey and the goop is hot and bubbly.

4. Serve with baby greens dressed with Makoto Dill Dressing.

TIP—You can use any fish of your choice, or even shrimp or a chicken breast. If you use a chicken breast, make sure the chicken is cooked through (see the roasting guide for poultry on page 310). These freeze beautifully in individual baking dishes for quick dinners. I always double the recipe to make 4 at a time: 2 for us and 2 for the freezer.

Chicken Cacciatore with Spaghetti Squash

Make this with your favorite low-SUGAR tomato sauce.

Ingredients
1 medium spaghetti squash (8 net carbs per cup)
2 tablespoons olive oil
1 cup cubed boneless, skinless chicken breast
½ cup chopped bell pepper (3 net carbs)
½ cup chopped mushrooms (2 net carbs)
¼ cup chopped onion (2.5 net carbs)
2 cloves garlic, minced (2 net carbs)
1 cup low-sugar pasta sauce (8 net carbs)
Salt and pepper
Grated Parmesan or Romano cheese

25.5 Net Carbs for entire recipe

1. Punch 10 or 12 steam vent holes about 2 inches deep into the spaghetti squash with a sharp knife. Place the spaghetti squash in the microwave and cook on high for about 20 minutes. To test doneness, gently squeeze with a gloved hand (it will be hot). If the squash gives, then it's done. If not, cook longer, checking at 5-minute intervals until it is soft enough to give when squeezed.

2. When the squash is done, place it on a cutting board and allow to cool for 10 minutes. Cut it in half lengthwise, then let stand to cool.

3. Heat the olive oil in a skillet over medium-high heat. Pan-fry the chicken breast cubes until nicely browned, then remove the chicken from the pan and set aside.

4. Add the bell pepper, mushrooms, onion, and garlic to the skillet and cook uncovered over medium-high heat for 5 minutes.

5. Add the pasta sauce and continue cooking. When it starts to bubble, add the chicken, cover, and reduce the heat to a simmer. After 5 minutes, remove from the heat and let rest.

6. With a fork, remove the seeds from the squash and discard. Now, using the fork, start pulling the squash meat out onto a plate. Notice that the meat looks like strands of angel hair pasta. Salt and pepper the squash to taste and toss with Romano or Parmesan cheese.

7. Once the squash is "dressed," transfer portions to dinner plates and smother with the cacciatore. Grate additional Romano or Parmesan cheese on top and serve.

Lasagna

Serves 2

Use your favorite low-SUGAR tomato sauce. Serve with a green salad.

Ingredients
2 tablespoons olive oil

½ pound ground beef
2 cloves garlic, minced (2 net carbs)
½ teaspoon Italian seasoning
Salt and pepper
1 cup ricotta cheese (8 net carbs)
1 cup shredded mozzarella cheese
1 large egg (1 net carb)
2 small zucchini (3 net carbs per cup)
1 cup low-sugar pasta sauce (8 net carbs)
Grated Parmesan or Romano cheese

22 Net Carbs for entire recipe

1. Preheat the oven to 350 degrees.

2. Heat the olive oil in a skillet over medium heat, then add the ground beef and garlic. Season with Italian seasoning and salt and pepper to taste. Cook until browned, then drain the fat and set aside.

3. In a mixing bowl, combine the ricotta cheese, ½ cup of the mozzarella cheese, and the egg. Salt and pepper to taste, mix well, and set aside.

4. Cut the zucchini into very thin lengthwise strips to take the place of lasagna noodles.

5. Spoon a couple tablespoons of your pasta sauce into the bottom of 2 individual baking dishes and add a couple of zucchini slices. Spoon on half of the cheese mixture as the next layer, sprinkle with a little more sauce, and layer on a couple of squash slices. Next, add a layer of meat and a little more sauce, then a couple more squash slices, topping it all with more sauce.

6. Sprinkle ¼ cup of the mozzarella cheese on top of each dish and bake for 30 minutes. All of your cheese should be melted and gooey.

7. Remove from the oven and cover with a good sprinkling of Parmesan or Romano cheese and serve.

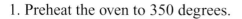

TIP—You can substitute Italian sausage or any ground meat (even a mixture of several) for the ground beef. These freeze beautifully in

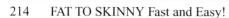

individual baking dishes for quick dinners. I always make 4 at a time: 2 for us and 2 for the freezer.

Seafood Bake

Serves 2

Buy scallops, shrimp, and your choice of fish from your local seafood market. (If you can't get fresh, frozen works well.)

Ingredients
2 tablespoons butter
½ pound scallops
½ pound shrimp, peeled and deveined
2 fish filets
Garlic salt
Ground pepper
Paprika

0 Net Carbs for entire recipe

1. Preheat the oven to 425 degrees.

2. In the microwave, melt a tablespoon of butter in each of 2 individual baking dishes. Divide the seafood into 2 portions and place one in each dish. Roll the seafood around in the butter to coat each side.

3. Arrange the seafood neatly in the dish and sprinkle with garlic salt, ground pepper, and paprika.

4. Bake for 15 minutes, or until the seafood is cooked through, and serve.

TIP—Freeze uncooked portions inside individual bakeware for a fast, easy dinner.

Shepherd's Pie

Ingredients
1 tablespoon olive oil
¾ pound ground beef
½ cup chopped onion (5 net carbs)
Salt and pepper
1 cup ricotta cheese (8 net carbs)
½ cup shredded cheddar cheese
½ cup shredded mozzarella cheese
1½ cups Caulimash, recipe on page 197 (4.5 net carbs)

17.5 Net Carbs for entire recipe

1. Preheat the oven to 350 degrees.

2. Heat the olive oil in a skillet. Cook the ground beef and onion until browned. Salt and pepper the beef to taste, then strain and set aside.

3. In a mixing bowl, combine the ricotta cheese, cheddar cheese, and mozzarella cheese.

4. Place half of the cooked ground beef and onion into a casserole dish. Layer on top of the meat half of the cheese mixture, then the Caulimash, then the remaining meat, and then cover all of it with a final layer of the remaining cheese.

5. Bake uncovered for 40 to 45 minutes, until heated through and the cheese is melted.

6. Using a large serving spoon, scoop one or two large spoonfuls of the casserole onto a dinner plate and serve.

Veal Parmesan with Spaghetti Squash

Ingredients
1 medium spaghetti squash (4 net carbs per ½ cup)
2 veal cutlets

1 large egg (1 net carb)
2 tablespoons heavy cream
¾ cup Fry Coating (recipe on page 251)
2 tablespoons olive oil
1 cup low-sugar pasta sauce (4 net carbs per ½ cup)
¾ cup shredded mozzarella cheese
Grated Parmesan or Romano cheese
Salt and pepper
Green salad (1.5 net carbs per cup)

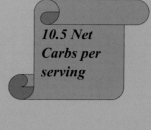

10.5 Net Carbs per serving

1. Punch 10 or 12 steam vent holes about 2 inches deep into the spaghetti squash with a knife. Place the spaghetti squash in the microwave and cook on high for about 20 minutes. To test doneness, gently squeeze with a gloved hand (it will be hot). If the squash gives, then it's done. If not, cook longer, checking at 5-minute intervals until it is soft enough to give when squeezed.

2. When the squash is done, place it on a cutting board and allow to cool for 10 minutes. Cut it in half lengthwise, then let stand to cool.

3. Beat the egg with the cream in a medium bowl. Pound the veal cutlets thin and place them in the egg wash, then dredge in the Fry Coating. Heat the olive oil in a skillet over medium-high heat and pan-fry the cutlets on both sides.

4. Cover the cutlets with the pasta sauce and mozzarella cheese and cover the pan to melt the cheese.

5. With a fork, remove the seeds from the squash and discard. Now, using the fork, start pulling the squash meat out onto a plate. Notice that the meat looks like strands of angel hair pasta. Salt and pepper the squash to taste and toss with Romano or Parmesan cheese.

6. Once the squash is "dressed," transfer portions to dinner plates. Remove cutlets from the pan and serve on top of the squash.

TIP—You can substitute a nice thin piece of fish, turkey, chicken cutlet, or eggplant for the veal.

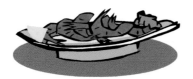

Baked Shrimp with Crabmeat Stuffing

Ingredients
1 cup lump crabmeat
1 large egg (1 net carb)
¼ cup chopped onion (2.5 net carbs)
¼ cup chopped green bell pepper (1.5 net carbs)
¼ cup shredded cheddar cheese
12–16 large shrimp
Butter
Salt and pepper
Green salad (add 1.5 net carbs per cup)

5 Net Carbs for entire recipe, minus green salad

1. Preheat the oven to 425 degrees.

2. In a mixing bowl, combine the crabmeat, egg, onion, green pepper, and cheddar cheese to make the stuffing.

3. Peel the shrimp, leaving the little tail end on. Using a sharp knife, butterfly the shrimp on the inside curve, opening the shrimp for stuffing.

4. Place the shrimp in a well-buttered baking dish side-by-side, with the tails facing up. Stuff each shrimp with a heaping teaspoon of stuffing, then season with salt and pepper to taste. Bake for 10 to 12 minutes, or until the shrimp is cooked through.

5. Serve with a green salad.

 TIP—Cook this recipe in individual baking dishes.

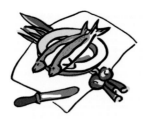

Triple Crown Baked Fish with Crabmeat Stuffing

I like grouper for this, but you can use another white fish of your choice.

Ingredients
1 cup lump crabmeat
1 large egg (1 net carb)
¼ cup chopped onion (2.5 net carbs)
¼ cup chopped green bell pepper (1.5 net carbs)
¼ cup shredded cheddar cheese
1 grouper filet or other white fish
1 salmon filet
Salt and pepper
Paprika
4 tablespoons butter plus a few additional pats
Sweet Lemon Caper Sauce, recipe follows
Green salad (add 1.5 net carbs per cup)

6 Net Carbs for entire recipe, minus green salad

1. Preheat the oven to 375 degrees.

2. Make the crabmeat stuffing as follows: In a mixing bowl, combine the crabmeat, egg, onion, green pepper, and cheddar cheese. Set aside.

3. Cut the white fish filet into 2 thin pieces. Cut the salmon filet into 2 thin pieces.

4. Place the white fish in the bottom of a well-buttered baking dish, layer in the crabmeat stuffing, and top with the salmon. Place butter pats on top of the fish and season with salt, pepper, and paprika to taste.

5. Bake for 20 to 25 minutes, or until the fish is cooked through.

6. Top with Sweet Lemon Caper Sauce. Serve with a green salad on the side.

Sweet Lemon Caper Sauce—Melt 4 tablespoons butter in the microwave. Add 1 tablespoon capers, 1 tablespoon lemon juice, and 1 teaspoon xylitol or stevia and stir to combine.

 TIP—Cook this recipe in individual baking dishes.

Salisbury Steak with Onions and Mushrooms over Mexican Caulimash

Serves 4

Ingredients
1 tablespoon olive oil
1 pound ground beef
½ cup sliced onion (1 net carb per ⅛ cup)
1 cup sliced mushrooms (4 net carbs)
1 cup Heinz Home Style Beef Gravy (4 net carbs per ¼ cup)

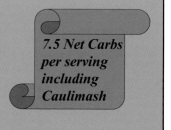

7.5 Net Carbs per serving including Caulimash

1. Heat the olive oil over medium-high heat in a nonstick skillet. Divide the beef into 4 hamburger patties and pan-fry.

2. While the burgers are cooking, toss the onion and mushrooms into the pan.

3. When you turn the burgers over, reduce the heat to low and pour in the gravy. Cover and simmer for 8 minutes.

4. Prepare the Mexican Caulimash as directed on page 198.

5. Serve the burgers and gravy over the Mexican Caulimash.

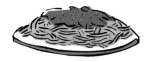

Chicken Parmesan with Spaghetti

Ingredients
2 boneless, skinless chicken breasts
1 large egg (1 net carb)
2 tablespoons heavy cream
¾ cup Fry Coating (recipe on page 251)
¼ cup olive oil
½ cup low-sugar pasta sauce (4 net carbs)
¾ cup shredded mozzarella cheese
1 package Tofu Shirataki Spaghetti or Fettuccini (2 net carbs)
Salt and pepper
Grated Parmesan or Romano cheese
Fresh basil leaves for garnish
Green salad (add 1.5 net carbs per cup)

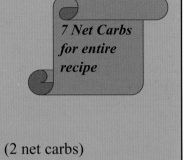

7 Net Carbs for entire recipe

1. Place a chicken breast in a quart-size zippered plastic bag and close the zipper 95 percent of the way. Place the bagged breast on the cutting board and, using a wine bottle or rolling pin, pound the breast thin.

2. Beat the egg with the cream in a medium bowl. Place a chicken breast in the egg wash and then dredge in Fry Coating. Repeat with the second breast.

3. Add the oil to a skillet and pan-fry the chicken on both sides over medium-high heat. When the breasts are cooked through, place them on a paper towel.

4. Carefully drain the remaining oil into a heat-proof container and wipe the pan clean with a paper towel.

5. Place the breasts back into the pan over medium-low heat. Put a couple of tablespoons of the pasta sauce on top of the cutlets, along with a handful of the mozzarella cheese, and cover to melt the cheese.

6. Rinse the noodles in a colander under very hot water, then drain.

7. Heat up the remaining pasta sauce in the microwave.

8. Once the noodles have drained, season with salt and pepper to taste and toss with Romano or Parmesan cheese and the hot pasta sauce.

9. When the pasta is dressed, transfer portions to dinner plates. Top with the cutlets, salt and pepper to taste, and garnish with fresh basil. Serve with green salad.

TIP—You can substitute a nice thin piece of fish, turkey cutlet, veal cutlet, or eggplant for the chicken.

Southern Fried Pork Chops with Green Beans, Shredded Cabbage, and Caulimash

Serves 4

Ingredients
1 large egg (1 net carb)
2 tablespoons heavy cream
4 pork chops
1 cup Fry Coating, recipe on page 251
¼ cup olive oil
2 cups green beans, trimmed (3 net carbs per ½ cup)
1½ tablespoons butter
2 cups shredded green cabbage (1.5 net carbs per ½ cup)

6 Net Carbs per serving including Caulimash

1. Beat the egg with the cream in a medium bowl. Place the chops in the egg wash, then dredge in the Fry Coating.

2. Pan-fry both sides of the chops in olive oil over medium heat, being careful not to burn them. The frying time will depend on the thickness of the chops. If the chops are very thick you may have to flip them a couple of times in order to cook them through without burning the coating. I like

chops around ½-inch thick, which cook quickly enough that only one flip is required.

3. While the chops are cooking, bring an inch of salted water to a boil in a saucepan over high heat. Cook the green beans to your desired tenderness and drain.

4. Using the same pot, melt a little butter in the bottom of the pot over medium-high heat and quickly stir-fry the cabbage to desired tenderness.

5. Prepare the Caulimash as directed on page 197.

6. Transfer the cabbage to a plate and cover with the green beans. Add the Caulimash and the chop. Add butter and salt and pepper to taste and serve.

Fried Chicken 'n' Strawberries with Sweet Sour Cream Dip

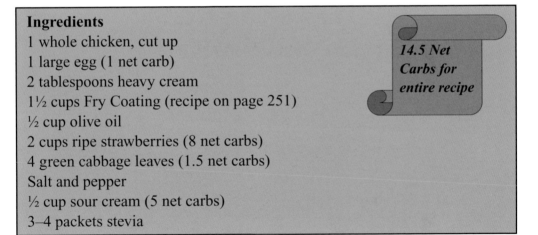

Ingredients
1 whole chicken, cut up
1 large egg (1 net carb)
2 tablespoons heavy cream
1½ cups Fry Coating (recipe on page 251)
½ cup olive oil
2 cups ripe strawberries (8 net carbs)
4 green cabbage leaves (1.5 net carbs)
Salt and pepper
½ cup sour cream (5 net carbs)
3–4 packets stevia

14.5 Net Carbs for entire recipe

1. Preheat the oven to 250 degrees. Set up a cookie sheet with a couple of paper towels spread on it and set aside.

2. Remove the skin from all the chicken parts. Beat the egg with the cream in a medium bowl. Place the chicken parts in the egg wash, then dredge in the Fry Coating.

3. Pan-fry both sides of the chicken pieces in olive oil over medium heat,

being careful not to burn. The length of time you fry the chicken will depend on the thickness of the parts. If the chicken parts are very thick you may have to flip them a couple of times in order to cook through without burning the coating. The wings will cook through first, the breast second, the thighs and legs last. Be careful not to overcook the breast as it will become dry.

4. While the chicken is cooking, prepare a serving plate by stripping a couple of large leaves from a cabbage head and arranging on the platter.

5. Clean the strawberries, leaving the leaves intact to be used as a handle for dipping them in the sweet sour cream dip (recipe follows). Arrange them on the serving platter.

6. As the chicken parts cook through and you remove them from the frying pan, place them on the paper-towel-lined cookie sheet and slip them into the oven to keep warm. When all of the chicken is cooked through, arrange the pieces on the platter, salt and pepper to taste, and serve.

Sweet Sour Cream Dip—There are two ways to serve this dip with the strawberries:

Method #1: Add a ½ cup of sour cream to a serving dish. Open 3 or 4 packets stevia and pile the sweetener beside the sour cream on the same plate. You first dip the strawberry into the sour cream and then into the pile of sweetener.

Method #2: Mix the sweetener into the sour cream until it reaches the desired sweetness. Place in a dipping bowl and arrange on the platter with the berries.

TIP—There's nothing better at a picnic than room-temperature fried chicken. Cook some extra pieces and go on a picnic this weekend . . . don't forget the deviled eggs!

Black and Blue Wasabi Tuna with Garlic Ginger Green Beans

Serves 2

Buy 2 nice yellowfin or blackfin tuna steaks from your local grocer or fish-monger. Smell them at the store; the odor should be very mild and not too "fishy."

Ingredients

2 fresh tuna steaks
2 tablespoons olive oil
1 teaspoon butter
½ teaspoon sesame oil
4 tablespoons sesame seeds (.5 net carb per 2
  tablespoons)
2 tablespoons 0-carb wasabi paste
1 cup green beans, trimmed (3 net carbs per ½ cup)
1 teaspoon minced fresh ginger
1 large garlic clove, minced (1 net carb)
Salt and pepper
2 tablespoons pickled ginger (2 net carbs)
Wasabi paste

6.5 Net Carbs per serving

1. Over medium-high heat, bring the beans and 1 inch of lightly salted water to a boil in a nonstick skillet. Cook the beans for 5 minutes, then strain.

2. Reduce the heat to low and return the skillet to the stove.

3. Melt the butter with the sesame oil in the pan. Sauté the minced ginger and minced garlic for 1 to 2 minutes, stirring constantly to avoid burning.

4. Toss in the beans and mix well to thoroughly coat them. Salt and pepper to taste and remove from the skillet.

5. Wipe out the skillet, increase the heat to medium-high, and add the olive oil.

6. Coat both sides of the fish heavily with sesame seeds (I prefer black seeds). The simplest way to do it is to spread the seeds onto a plate and press the fish into the seeds.

7. Cook the fish in the hot oil no more than 12 seconds for each side, and remove from the heat. The fish should be very pink inside when sliced.

8. Serve with wasabi paste, pickled ginger, and a side of green beans.

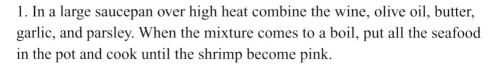 **TIP**—You can find sweetened or unsweetened pickled ginger in your local store. I buy the unsweetened variety and add a couple of packets stevia or xylitol to the bottle, keeping it sugar-free.

Snow Crab and Shrimp in White Wine–Garlic Sauce

Serves 4

Buy the shrimp and snow crab clusters from your local fishmonger.

Ingredients
4 large snow crab clusters
1½ pounds large shrimp
2 cups white wine
¼ cup olive oil
4 tablespoons butter
6 large cloves of garlic, minced (6 net carbs)
2 tablespoons chopped fresh parsley (1.5 net carbs)

7.5 Net Carbs for entire recipe

1. In a large saucepan over high heat combine the wine, olive oil, butter, garlic, and parsley. When the mixture comes to a boil, put all the seafood in the pot and cook until the shrimp become pink.

2. Remove the pot from the stove and scoop out all the seafood onto a serving platter. Coat the seafood with a ladle-full of liquid from the pot and serve. Accompany each serving with small dishes of the sauce for dipping.

3. Serve with a veggie tray (see page 127) and salad dressing dips (remember to add the additional carbs).

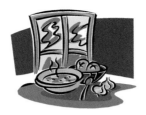

Shrimp Gumbo Filé

Serves 6

Ingredients
2 tablespoons olive oil
2 boneless, skinless chicken breasts, cut into 1-inch cubes
1 package Hillshire Farm Light Smoked Sausage, sliced
1 cup chopped celery (3 net carbs)
1 cup chopped green bell pepper (6 net carbs)
½ cup chopped onion (5 net carbs)
4 cloves garlic, crushed (4 net carbs)
8 cups canned no-sugar chicken broth
2–4 tablespoons Cajun Land Cajun Seasoning
1 cup okra (6 net carbs)
1½ pounds large shrimp, shelled and deveined
1½ pounds cod filets, cut into 1-inch cubes
2 teaspoons filé powder (ground sassafras)

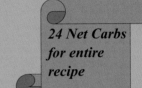

24 Net Carbs for entire recipe

1. For the gumbo, heat the olive oil in the bottom of a stewpot. Add the chicken, sausage, celery, green pepper, onion, and garlic and cook until browned.

2. Pour in the chicken broth. Bring to a boil and add the Cajun seasoning and sliced okra (thawed out from the freezer is okay). Reduce the heat to low and simmer for 20 minutes.

3. Now it's time to taste the broth. Is it spicy enough, salty enough? If not, add another couple teaspoons of Cajun seasoning, stir, and taste again. Continue to adjust seasonings until your desired spice level is achieved.

4. Add the shrimp and fish to the pot, cover, and simmer another 10 minutes.

5. Just prior to serving, sprinkle the filé powder on top of the stew pot and gently mix in.

6. Serve with Jalapeño-Cheddar Cheese Cornbread (recipe follows).

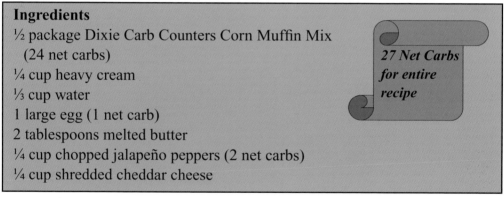

TIP—The gumbo freezes well for quick soup-and-salad lunch. If you wish to make a smaller batch, simply cut all the ingredient quantities in half.

Jalapeño-Cheddar Cheese Cornbread

Dixie Carb Counters Corn Muffin Mix is available at **www.dixiediner.com**.

Ingredients
½ package Dixie Carb Counters Corn Muffin Mix
   (24 net carbs)
¼ cup heavy cream
⅓ cup water
1 large egg (1 net carb)
2 tablespoons melted butter
¼ cup chopped jalapeño peppers (2 net carbs)
¼ cup shredded cheddar cheese

27 Net Carbs for entire recipe

1. Preheat the oven to 400 degrees. Grease a 6-muffin pan or pie dish with nonstick cooking spray.

2. Mix the corn muffin mix with the cream, water, egg, and butter.

3. Add the jalapeños and cheddar cheese.

4. Pour into the prepared pan and place in the oven to bake for 12 minutes.

Pork Chops Marsala with Caulimash

Serves 2

Ingredients
1 tablespoon olive oil
1 cup whole mushrooms (4 net carbs)
½ cup marsala (2 net carbs)
Salt and pepper
2 pork chops, 1 inch thick
½ cup thinly sliced yellow onion (5 net carbs)
1 tablespoon butter

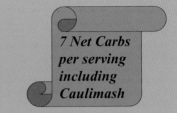

7 Net Carbs per serving including Caulimash

1. Heat the olive oil in a skillet over medium-high heat. While the pan is heating, marinate the mushrooms in ¼ cup of the marsala.

2. Salt and pepper both sides of the pork chops. Place the chops in the skillet and brown one side. Flip the chops over and wait 60 seconds, then pour in the mushrooms and marsala. Add the onion. Cover the pan and reduce the heat to medium-low. Cook for 15 minutes.

3. Meanwhile, make the Caulimash according to the recipe on page 197.

4. After you've cooked the pork for 15 minutes, remove the chops and vegetables to a serving plate, leaving the remaining liquid in the pan. Raise the heat to medium-high and add the butter and the remaining ¼ cup marsala to the pan. Reduce the liquid to a creamy texture and drizzle over the chops.

5. Serve the chops over Caulimash.

Paella

Ingredients
1 head cauliflower, trimmed and cut into chunks (1.5 net carbs per ½ cup)
4 tablespoons butter or Benecol spread, melted
Salt and pepper
3 slices yellow onion (2 net carbs)

1 medium red bell pepper, sliced (3 net carbs)
1 boneless, skinless chicken breast
2 raw Italian sausage links (2 net carbs)
1 salmon filet
6 medium or large shrimp
6 large scallops
Dill weed
Italian seasoning

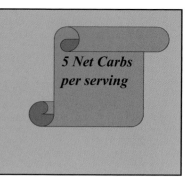

5 Net Carbs
per serving

1. Prepare cauliflower "rice" (Cauli-rice) by processing a head of cauliflower in a food processor with a chopping blade until it resembles rice. Add 3 tablespoons of the melted butter or Benecol spread. Salt and pepper to taste, then mix well.

2. Preheat the oven to 400 degrees. Generously butter a shallow casserole or baking dish (my favorite is my 10-inch cast iron frying pan with a self-basting cover).

3. Transfer the "rice" to the bottom of the baking dish. Place the onion and sliced pepper on top of the rice as if you were making a pizza.

4. Slice the chicken breast and sausage into ½-inch slices and arrange on top. Cut the salmon into 2-inch squares and arrange the salmon, shrimp, and scallops throughout the dish.

5. Sprinkle the remaining 1 tablespoon melted butter all over the ingredients and season with dill weed, Italian seasoning, and salt and pepper to taste. Cover the baking dish and bake for 45 minutes.

6. When serving, measure out the Cauli-rice and plate it by spreading it over the surface of the dish. Place veggies, meat, and seafood on top of the Cauli-rice and salt and pepper to taste.

Hawaiian Luau Spare Ribs with Wasabi Coleslaw

The key to this recipe is marinade time, the longer the better. I usually marinate my ribs in a gallon-size zippered plastic bag for 48 hours prior to cooking. You *can* marinate for half the time, however the ribs won't have as "rich" a flavor.

Ingredients
4–6 country-style pork ribs
½ cup Crystal Light Orange Pineapple drink mix
¼ cup soy sauce (4 net carbs)
¼ cup sugar-free teriyaki sauce
½ cup chopped white onion (5 net carbs)
2 tablespoons black and white sesame seeds
4 cloves garlic, minced (4 net carbs)

13 Net Carbs for entire recipe

1. Trim the excess fat off the ribs and set aside.

2. In a gallon-size zippered plastic bag, combine the drink mix, soy sauce, teriyaki sauce, onion, sesame seeds, and garlic. Place the ribs in the marinade and swish around until all the meat is well coated. Seal the bag and place in the fridge on a plate for 2 days.

3. Preheat the grill to medium heat.

4. Take out the ribs and place them on the grill, reserving the remaining marinade to be used as a basting sauce. Cook the ribs with the lid closed. (See the grilling chart for pork on page 306 for cooking times.)

5. When it's time to flip the ribs, generously baste with the remaining liquid. Close the lid and finish the cooking process. If flare-ups occur, reduce the heat a bit. Continue cooking until cooked through.

6. Serve with Wasabi Coleslaw (recipe follows).

Wasabi Sesame Coleslaw

Ingredients
2 packed cups shredded green cabbage (6 net carbs)
Salt and pepper
2 tablespoons Kraft Green Goddess Dressing (2 net carbs)

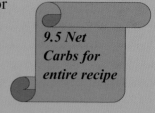

9.5 Net Carbs for entire recipe

Place the cabbage in a mixing bowl, and salt and pepper to taste. In a separate bowl, mix the green goddess dressing, wasabi mustard, sour cream, mayonnaise, vinegar, sesame seeds, and stevia. Add the dressing to the cabbage and mix well. Let stand at least 1 hour prior to serving.

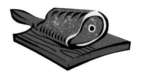

Roast Prime Rib of Beef with French Onion Soup

This is my dad's favorite meal. He loves a nice piece of prime rib and strawberry shortcake for dessert. He couldn't care less if he had anything else on his plate. ☺

Prime rib can be fairly expensive, so some advance preparation should be taken. Here are the questions that need to be answered: how big a roast, how many people are we serving, and how long do you cook it? On page TK[x-ref], you'll find the charts I've prepared for you to answer those questions. Remember, the more well done the meat is, the tougher it will be. Personally, I prefer my roast rare—it will melt in your mouth. Serve with French Onion Soup, recipe follows.

Ingredients
6–8 pound prime rib roast (3 ribs)
Coarsely ground salt and pepper

0 Net Carbs for entire recipe without soup

1. Whichever size roast you buy, a few rules pertain to all. First, make sure the roast has reached room temperature all the way through. Simply leave the fully defrosted roast on the counter until temperature is reached. Next,

you'll need a very hot oven, 450 degrees, to begin the cooking process. Preheat the oven and let's prep the meat.

2. If the roast has a layer of fat on top more than ½ inch thick, you'll want to trim off the excess fat. Simply take a sharp chef's knife and run it across the top of the roast, cutting away the excess fat but leaving between ¼ inch and ½ inch intact. It's the fat that will self-baste the roast. Once the roast is trimmed, generously sprinkle with coarse salt and pepper.

3. Place the roast in a shallow baking pan (I like to use a cast iron skillet) and place the pan in the hot preheated oven. Cook at high heat for 15 minutes, then reduce the heat to 325 degrees for the remainder of the cooking time. I suggest you buy a good meat thermometer. They are not expensive and they will keep you out of trouble. Check the meat's internal temperature about three-quarters of the way through the cooking time (see chart on page 298) by sticking the thermometer into the center of the roast. Ovens vary in temperature, so it's a good idea to keep an eye on it.

4. While your roast is cooking, let's prepare your French onion soup. Go through all the steps in the recipe that follows and stop at the point where you place the cheese on top of the crocks. Your soup will only be in the oven for a couple of minutes under the broiler, so you'll want to melt your cheese just prior to serving your roast. If your soup was prepared in advance and has cooled, heat each crock in the microwave prior to topping with the cheese and placing in the oven.

5. Once the roast has reached the proper temperature, remove it from the oven and let stand 15 to 20 minutes prior to carving. Letting the roast stand allows the juices to coagulate and not run out of the roast, which would leave it dry. As mentioned, I like my prime rib rare.

6. To carve the roast, run your knife along the ribs first and cut them away. Then you can cut smaller slices without interference from the bones. Place the side of the roast from which you removed the ribs flat on your cutting board, leaving the fat side up. Using a sharp carving knife and a carving fork, slice off the appropriate serving sizes. Plate and serve with French onion soup.

French Onion Soup

Serves 4

Avoid the little cubes of dried bouillon: they are full of salt and not very flavorful. You can buy higher quality products, including bouillon (also known as broth) in a carton. You will need 4 individual-size crocks or oven-proof bowls.

Ingredients
2 large sweet onions (20 net carbs)
2 tablespoons butter, plus extra to grease crocks
5 cups beef broth
4 teaspoons Worcestershire sauce (4 net carbs)
Salt and pepper
4 slices Swiss cheese (long slices)

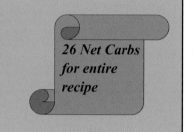

26 Net Carbs for entire recipe

1. Slice the onions into ¼-inch slices, then cut those slices in half.

2. Melt the butter in a medium saucepan over medium-high heat and sauté the onions until they begin to caramelize. The process of caramelizing simply brings out the natural sugars in the onions. They will be wilted and a nice brown color. This will take a bit of time, as long as ten minutes, so be patient and stir often.

3. Now, add the beef broth and Worcestershire sauce. Taste for seasoning and add salt and pepper if necessary, and bring to a boil. Remove from the heat.

4. Using a ladle, distribute equal amounts of broth into each of 4 crocks. Then divide the onions among the crocks.

5. Using a stick of butter, grease the inside lip and outside lip of the crocks to make for easy cleaning. Cut each long slice of cheese in half. Lay 2 pieces over the top of the crock in a cross ("+").

6. Place the crocks on a cookie sheet in the oven on a high rack. Broil until the cheese is melted. Remove immediately from the oven and serve.

Korean Baby Back Ribs with Wasabi Coleslaw

The key to this recipe is marinating time. I usually marinate my ribs for 24 hours, prior to cooking, in a large zippered plastic bag.

Ingredients
½ cup soy sauce (8 net carbs)
½ cup sugar-free teriyaki sauce
½ cup chopped scallions (2.5 net carbs)
¼ cup garlic oil
5 large cloves garlic, chopped (5 net carbs)
2 tablespoons black and white sesame seeds
2 tablespoons finely chopped fresh ginger (1.5 net carbs)
1 teaspoon powdered ginger
4 or 5 packets stevia or xylitol
1 rack pork spare ribs
Cracked black pepper

12.5 Net Carbs for entire recipe

1. In the bag, mix the soy sauce, teriyaki sauce, scallions, garlic oil, garlic, sesame seeds, fresh ginger, powdered ginger, and stevia or xylitol.

2. Place the ribs in the bag and swish around until all the meat is well coated. Close the bag and place in the fridge in a large bowl for 24 hours.

3. When the ribs are done marinating, preheat the oven to 325 degrees.

4. Put the ribs and all the marinade in a baking dish. Grind a good helping of black pepper over the ribs.

5. Cover with foil and bake for 3½ hours. Uncover the ribs and finish the last 30 minutes of cooking uncovered.

6. Serve with Wasabi Sesame Coleslaw (recipe on page 250).

 TIP—The key to good ribs is to cook them slow and low.

Video-supported recipe! Go to this Web site to watch me make it for you: **www.FATtoSKINNY.com/recipes.htm.**

Bacon Burger in a Kale Blanket

Ingredients
6–8 kale leaves (7 net carbs)
3 slices bacon, chopped
1 cup oil-marinated artichoke hearts, drained (4 net carbs)
1 cup diced eggplant (4 net carbs)
4 celery stalks, chopped (3 net carbs)
¼ cup chopped onion (2.5 net carbs)
1 pound ground beef
2 cups shredded mozzarella cheese
Nonstick cooking spray
Salt and pepper
1 cup low-sugar marinara sauce (8 net carbs)
6 slices provolone cheese (optional)

28.5 Net Carbs for entire recipe

1. Parboil the kale in lightly salted boiling water for 15 minutes. Drain the leaves and let cool for a few minutes.

2. Preheat the oven to 375 degrees. Coat a glass baking dish with nonstick cooking spray.

3. Using the same pot that you used for the kale, pan-fry the bacon. When the bacon is browned, add the artichoke hearts, eggplant, celery, and onion. Cook over medium-high heat until all the ingredients are slightly browned.

4. Turn off the heat; add the ground beef and shredded mozzarella cheese. Mix all the ingredients together with a pinch of salt and pepper and set aside.

5. On a cutting board, use a sharp knife to slice the largest part of each kale stem away from the thin leafy part creating a "^" shape in the bottom of the leaf.

6. Fill each of the kale leaves with a scoop of filling, folding down the top of the leaf first, then folding each of the bottom ends up, closing the leaf. Flip the packet over and place in the baking dish. Repeat these steps until the baking dish is full.

7. Spread the marinara sauce over the stuffed leaves. Cover the dish with aluminum foil and bake for 1 hour, or until the leaves are fork tender and everything is heated through. At 50 minutes you can uncover the dish and add provolone cheese to the top and broil for 10 more minutes if you want a more savory dish.

8. Scoop out a burger or two from the dish, plate, and serve.

Crabby Face-Off

You can use canned crabmeat for this recipe. Adding caviar brings an additional savory side to any seafood dish. It's a bit expensive, but a little goes a long way. Caviar is very salty, so adjust your salt accordingly.

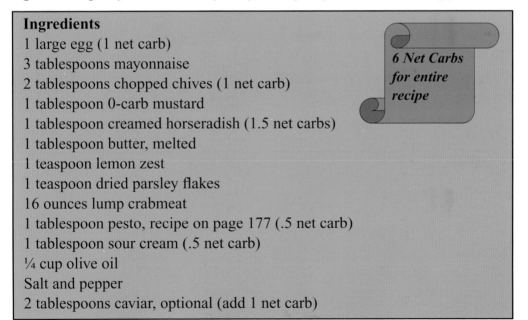

Ingredients
1 large egg (1 net carb)
3 tablespoons mayonnaise
2 tablespoons chopped chives (1 net carb)
1 tablespoon 0-carb mustard
1 tablespoon creamed horseradish (1.5 net carbs)
1 tablespoon butter, melted
1 teaspoon lemon zest
1 teaspoon dried parsley flakes
16 ounces lump crabmeat
1 tablespoon pesto, recipe on page 177 (.5 net carb)
1 tablespoon sour cream (.5 net carb)
¼ cup olive oil
Salt and pepper
2 tablespoons caviar, optional (add 1 net carb)

6 Net Carbs for entire recipe

1. In a large mixing bowl, combine the egg, 2 tablespoons mayonnaise, chives, mustard, horseradish, butter, lemon zest, and parsley. Whisk all

ingredients together well, then fold in the crabmeat very carefully so as to not break up the larger pieces. Cover with plastic wrap and place in the refrigerator overnight to develop the flavors.

2. Combine the pesto, sour cream, and the remaining tablespoon of mayonnaise. Whisk together to make the topping, then cover and place in the fridge.

3. The next day, heat the olive oil in a nonstick skillet over medium-high heat. Gently make patties with the crab mixture, being careful not to overwork. When the oil is hot, pan-fry the patties until they are golden brown on both sides.

4. Remove the patties to serving plates and and season with salt and pepper to taste. Spoon a dollop of topping on each cake and crown with caviar if desired.

Creamed Curry Sausage Bake

Ingredients
6 links Hillshire Farm Light Smoked Sausage
1 cup diced jicama (5 net carbs)
1 cup broccoli florets (4 net carbs)
1 cup diced zucchini (3 net carbs)
2 tablespoons olive oil
2 tablespoons dried green curry seasoning
1 cup Rich and Creamy Alfredo Sauce, recipe on page 167 (1 net carb)

13 Net Carbs for entire recipe

1. Preheat the oven to 400 degrees.

2. Cut the smoked sausage into ½-inch slices and place in a large mixing bowl. Dice the jicama, zucchini, and broccoli florets, then add to the sausage. Drizzle the olive oil and dried green curry seasoning over the mixture and incorporate all the ingredients evenly.

3. Spread the mixture onto a lipped cookie sheet in a single layer and bake for 20 minutes.

4. Heat up the Alfredo sauce until slightly simmering, then add the baked sausage and vegetables to the sauce and toss to coat. Transfer to a serving plate and enjoy.

TIP—If you want the jicama to taste more like diced potatoes, simmer them on the stove for an hour before using them in the recipe above. They will be slightly more tender.

Greek Sea Scallops with Fettuccini Alfredo and Baked Pesto Broccoli

Ingredients
1 pound large sea scallops, thawed if frozen
1 cup Blue Diamond Almond Breeze unsweetened vanilla almond milk
1 cup broccoli florets (4 net carbs)
2 tablespoons grated Romano cheese
1 tablespoon pesto, recipe on page 177 (.5 net carb)
2 tablespoons olive oil
¼ teaspoon sea salt
1 teaspoon salt
1 teaspoon garlic powder
1 teaspoon onion powder
1 tablespoon cooking sherry
1 package Tofu Shirataki Fettuccini (2 net carbs)
1 cup Rich and Creamy Alfredo Sauce, recipe on page 167 (1 net carb)

7.5 Net Carbs for entire recipe

1. Soak the scallops in the almond milk for 4 hours to enhance the flavor and plump up the scallops. Drain the scallops and set aside.

2. Preheat the oven to 350 degrees.

3. Combine the broccoli in a mixing bowl with the Romano cheese, pesto, 1 tablespoon of olive oil, and sea salt. Mix well. Spread the mixture on a cookie sheet and place in the preheated oven; cook for 20 minutes. While the broccoli is cooking, prepare the scallops.

4. Mix the salt, onion powder, and garlic powder together and add to the drained scallops; toss carefully to coat evenly.

5. Heat the remaning olive oil in a skillet over medium-high heat. Pan-fry the scallops until well seared on each side.

6. Add the sherry to the pan to deglaze the scallops, then remove the cooked scallops to a serving plate.

7. Rinse the noodles well and drain in a colander. Add the noodles and the Alfredo sauce to the scallop pan. Cook for a few more minutes until well heated, to combine the flavors.

8. Serve the Alfredo noodles onto the plate with the scallops and broccoli; enjoy.

TIP—Frozen scallops can be used, but be careful of the moisture content. Scallops should be cooked for a minimum amount of time and start off in the pan as dry as possible to get a nice sear.

Sweet 'n' Spicy Hickory Smoked Ribs

Purchase a meaty rack of fresh pork spare ribs for this dish.

Ingredients
1 rack pork spare ribs
½ cup xylitol
3 tablespoons hickory smoke rub
3 tablespoons smoked paprika
1 tablespoon chipotle powder
1 tablespoon onion powder
1 tablespoon garlic powder
1 tablespoon dried thyme
1 tablespoon chili powder
1 teaspoon salt
1 teaspoon white pepper

0 Net Carbs for entire recipe

1. Preheat the oven to 325 degrees with a rack in the center.

2. Place the ribs in a large baking pan.

3. In a small bowl, whisk together the xylitol, hickory smoke rub, smoked paprika, chipotle powder, onion powder, garlic powder, dried thyme, chili powder, salt, and white pepper. Rub a heavy coat of the mixture into the rib meat on both sides.

4. Pour ¼ cup water into the corner of the baking dish with the ribs and cover the dish well with aluminum foil.

5. Bake for 3 hours or until the meat pulls away easily from the bone with a fork. Let cool for 10 minutes. Finish on a heated grill for 10 to 15 minutes to char the edges.

TIP—If you double the recipe, adjust the bake time by another hour. These ribs freeze extremely well.

Bombay Shrimp with Coconut Gravy

Ingredients
1 teaspoon minced fresh ginger
1 teaspoon garlic powder
½ teaspoon salt
½ teaspoon cayenne pepper
¼ teaspoon turmeric
¼ teaspoon chili powder
24 large raw shrimp, peeled and deveined
2 tablespoons olive oil
½ cup coconut milk (2 net carbs)
1 tablespoon finely chopped fresh cilantro (1 net carb)

3 Net Carbs for entire recipe

1. Mix together the ginger, garlic powder, salt, cayenne, turmeric, and chili powder. Pour the seasonings over the shrimp and mix well to thoroughly coat the shrimp. Set aside for 10 minutes.

2. Heat the olive oil in a cast iron skillet over high heat. Sear both sides of the shrimp, about 1½ minutes on each side. Reduce the heat to medium and add the coconut milk and cilantro. Simmer for 3 to 4 minutes, or until the gravy thickens. Remove the shrimp from the heat.

3. Serve with a green salad tossed with a low-carb dressing (be sure to take the extra carbs from the salad and dressing into account for your net daily carb intake).

Italian Scallop Scampi

Ingredients
2 pounds large bay scallops
1 cup Blue Diamond Almond Breeze unsweetened
  vanilla almond milk (1 net carb)
2 tablespoons Italian seasoning
2 tablespoons olive oil
5 cloves garlic , minced (5 net carbs)
2 tablespoons butter
½ cup white wine (1 net carb)
2 cups broccoli florets (8 net carbs)
1 cup canned artichoke hearts, drained (4 net carbs)
2 tablespoons grated Romano cheese

17 Net Carbs for entire recipe

1. Soak the scallops in the almond milk overnight. Drain very well for an hour in a strainer in the fridge.

2. When the scallops are dry, rub them with Italian seasoning.

3. Heat the olive oil in a large cast iron skillet over high heat and add the garlic, then add the seasoned scallops. Cook for 2 minutes on the first side, then drop a few teaspoons of butter into the pan and flip the scallops, cooking for an additional 2 minutes.

4. Deglaze the pan by pouring ¼ cup white wine into the skillet and simmer the scallops for 1 more minute.

5. Scoop out scallops to a serving plate. Pour the sauce into individual ramekins.

6. Add a tablespoon of butter to the heated cast iron skillet (do not clean the pan) and toss in the broccoli and artichoke hearts. Sauté for about 5 minutes to heat through. Add the grated Romano cheese to the mixture while constantly stirring. Deglaze the pan once again with ¼ cup of white wine and simmer for an additional minute.

7. Serve the scallops with the broccoli and artichokes.

TIP—The trick to searing scallops is to make sure the heat is very high and the moisture content is minimal. If the heat is too low or you didn't drain them well enough, then the scallops will simply sweat and make a soup, shrinking in size all the while. But if you sear them properly, the juices remain in the scallop and a nice brown toasted crust will form.

Carnivore Pizza

Serves 2

Light Lavash Bread is available at **www.samisbakery.com**.

Ingredients
1 piece Light Lavash Bread (16 net carbs)
3 tablespoons pesto, recipe on page 177 (1.5 net carbs)
¼ cup stewed tomatoes, drained and chopped (1.5 net carbs)
¾ teaspoon Italian seasoning
½ packet stevia
½ teaspoon red pepper flakes, optional
1 cup shredded low-moisture mozzarella cheese or
   fresh mozzarella cheese, sliced
¼ cup chopped cooked chicken breast
¼ cup chopped ham
¼ cup sliced pepperoni

19 Net Carbs for entire recipe

1. Preheat the oven to 400 degrees with a pizza stone on the center rack.

2. Spread the pesto over the lavash and cover with the stewed tomatoes. Sprinkle the tomatoes with the Italian seasoning and stevia. Add red pepper flakes if you desire heat.

3. Cover with the shredded mozzarella cheese or slices of fresh mozzarella cheese if desired. Add chopped chicken, ham, and pepperoni.

4. Carefully slip the pizza onto the preheated pizza stone in the oven. Bake for 12 minutes, or until the edges of the lavash are golden brown and crispy.

5. Remove from the oven using a pizza peel and slice into 8 pieces (4 slices per serving).

Beef Enchiladas with Sour Cream and Guacamole

Serves 6

Ingredients
1½ pounds ground beef
½ cup chopped onion (5 net carbs)
2 tablespoons minced jalapeño pepper, plus
  sliced jalapeño for garnish, optional (1 net carb)
2 cups shredded cheddar cheese
1 cup low-sugar enchilada sauce (12 net carbs)
Nonstick cooking spray
6 La Tortilla Factory tortillas (18 net carbs)
6 tablespoons guacamole, recipe on page 184
  (3 net carbs)
6 tablespoons sour cream (3.5 net carbs)
6 cups salad greens (6 net carbs)
Hot sauce, optional

8 Net Carbs per serving

1. Preheat the oven to 400 degrees.

2. Brown the ground beef in a skillet.

3. Combine the onion, chopped jalapeño pepper (if desired), and 1⅓ cups of the cheese in a bowl.

4. When the beef is cooked, drain the fat and add the beef to the onion-pepper-cheese mixture. Add half of the enchilada sauce to thoroughly moisten the mixture, then set aside and let cool. Remove ½ cup of the filling to be used as a topping.

5. Spray a large casserole or individual casseroles with nonstick cooking spray. Lightly coat the bottom of the baking dish with enchilada sauce and set aside.

6. Place 3 heaping tablespoons of the filling into the center of a tortilla, then roll up and place, seam down, in the casserole dish. Repeat with the remaining tortillas and filling. Sprinkle the reserved filling across the top of the enchiladas and generously coat with the remaining enchilada sauce. Top the dish off with the remaining cheese and bake uncovered for 30 minutes, or until the cheese is melted and bubbly and the dish is heated through.

7. Portion the salad greens on each plate and serve the enchiladas on top. Add a tablespoon of sour cream and a tablespoon of guacamole. Garnish with a couple of slices of jalapeño pepper and serve with hot sauce if desired.

TIP—You can use many different filling replacements for the beef. Chicken, shrimp, turkey, or even cubed tofu for you vegans out there. All work well as enchilada fillings.

Stuffed Mexican Cabbage Bake on Cauli-rice with Sour Cream and Guacamole

Serves 6

Ingredients
1 teaspoon salt
6 large green cabbage leaves (4 net carbs)
1½ pounds ground beef
½ cup chopped onion (5 net carbs)

6.5 Net Carbs per serving

2 tablespoons minced jalapeño pepper, optional
   (1 net carb)
2 cups shredded cheddar cheese
1 cup low-sugar enchilada sauce (12 net carbs)
Nonstick cooking spray
3 cups Cauli-rice, recipe follows (9 net carbs)
6 tablespoons guacamole, recipe on page 184 (3 net carbs)
6 tablespoons sour cream (3.5 net carbs)
Hot sauce, optional

1. Bring 2 quarts water to a boil in a large pot; add the salt.

2. Carefully peel off 6 cabbage leaves from a large head of green cabbage and place them in the boiling water for 6 minutes. Drain the cabbage leaves and rinse with cool water; leave in a strainer in the sink.

3. Preheat the oven to 400 degrees.

4. Brown the ground beef in a skillet.

5. Combine the onion, chopped jalapeño pepper (if desired), and 1⅓ cups of the cheese in a mixing bowl.

6. When the beef is cooked, drain the fat and add the beef to the bowl with the onion, pepper, and cheese. Add half of the enchilada sauce to thoroughly moisten the mixture, then set aside and let cool. Remove ½ cup of the filling to be used as a topping.

7. Spray a large casserole or individual casseroles with nonstick cooking spray. Lightly coat the bottom with enchilada sauce and set aside.

8. Lay out a cabbage leaf on the cutting board. If the leaf has a thick stem at the bottom, trim off that section, about an inch up the leaf. This will make the leaf a uniform thickness and make it easier to roll. Place 3 heaping tablespoons of the filling into the center of the leaf, then roll up and place, seam down, in the casserole dish. Repeat with the remaining cabbage leaves and filling.

9. Sprinkle the reserved filling across the top of the cabbage rolls and

generously coat with the remaining enchilada sauce. Top the dish off with the remaining cheese and bake uncovered for 30 minutes, or until the cabbage is fork-tender, the cheese is melted, and the dish is heated through.

10. Spread the Cauli-rice out on serving plates and place the cabbage rolls on top. Add a tablespoon of sour cream and a tablespoon of guacamole to each serving. Garnish with a couple of slices of jalapeño pepper and serve with hot sauce if desired.

TIP—These rolls freeze well. Make extra servings in individual baking dishes and freeze unbaked, wrapped in plastic wrap, for a quick, easy meal.

Cauli-rice

Ingredients
1 head cauliflower, trimmed and cut into chunks
  (1.5 net carbs per ½ cup)
1 tablespoon butter
1 teaspoon salt
½ teaspoon ground black pepper

1.5 Net Carbs per ½ cup serving

Process a head of cauliflower in a food processor with a shredder blade until the cauliflower resembles rice. Remove to a mixing bowl, add the salt and pepper, and mix well. Melt the butter in a nonstick skillet over medium heat. Stir-fry the Cauli-rice to your desired doneness.

TIP—You can use many different spices in this wonderful rice replacement. Try chopped fresh basil or tarragon for a unique twist.

Stuffed Italian Cabbage Rolls 'n' Noodles

Serves 6

Ingredients
1 teaspoon salt

6 large green cabbage leaves (4 net carbs)
1½ pounds ground pork
1 cup uncooked Cauli-rice, recipe on page 247
  (3 net carbs)
1 cup shredded Fontina cheese
½ cup chopped onion (5 net carbs)
1 cup low-sugar pasta sauce (8 net carbs)
Nonstick cooking spray
2 cups shredded mozzarella cheese
3 packages Tofu Shirataki Fettuccini or Spaghetti (6 net carbs)
1 tablespoon extra-virgin olive oil
8 tablespoons grated Romano or Parmesan cheese
1 teaspoon pepper
1 teaspoon Italian seasoning

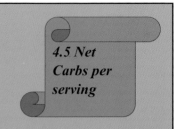

4.5 Net Carbs per serving

1. Bring 2 quarts water to a boil in a large pot; add the salt.

2. Carefully peel off 6 cabbage leaves from a large head of green cabbage and place them in the boiling water for 6 minutes. Drain the cabbage leaves and rinse with cool water; leave in strainer in sink.

3. Preheat the oven to 375 degrees.

4. Brown the ground pork in a skillet.

5. Combine the Cauli-rice, Fontina cheese, and onion in a mixing bowl; mix well.

6. When the pork is cooked, drain the fat and add the pork to the Cauli-rice mixture. Add half of the pasta sauce to thoroughly moisten the mixture, then set aside and let cool.

7. Spray a large casserole or individual casseroles with nonstick cooking spray. Lightly coat the bottom with pasta sauce and set aside.

8. Lay out a cabbage leaf on the cutting board. If the leaf has a thick stem at the bottom, trim off that section, about an inch up the leaf. This will make the leaf a uniform thickness and make it easier to roll. Place 3 to 4 heaping tablespoons

of the filling into the center of the leaf, then roll up and place, seam down, in the casserole dish. Repeat with the remaining cabbage leaves and filling.

9. Sprinkle the remaining filling and pasta sauce over the top of the cabbage rolls and cover with the mozzarella cheese. Bake uncovered for 30 minutes, or until the cabbage is fork-tender, the cheese is melted, and the dish is heated through.

10. Rinse the noodles well under hot water. Drain and pat dry with paper towels. Place the noodles into a mixing bowl and add olive oil, Romano or Parmesan cheese, Italian seasoning, and pepper. Mix well and set aside.

11. Serve the cabbage rolls on top of the noodles spread out on a plate. Top them off with more Romano or Parmesan cheese.

TIP—These rolls freeze well. Make extra servings in individual baking dishes and freeze unbaked, wrapped in plastic wrap, for a quick, easy meal.

Fried Fish with Wasabi Coleslaw

Buy your favorite fish filets from your grocer or fishmonger. Try to keep the filets no more than ¾ to 1 inch thick. This way the filet will cook through quickly without burning and will retain its crunch.

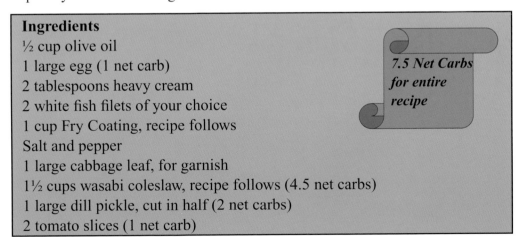

Ingredients
½ cup olive oil
1 large egg (1 net carb)
2 tablespoons heavy cream
2 white fish filets of your choice
1 cup Fry Coating, recipe follows
Salt and pepper
1 large cabbage leaf, for garnish
1½ cups wasabi coleslaw, recipe follows (4.5 net carbs)
1 large dill pickle, cut in half (2 net carbs)
2 tomato slices (1 net carb)

7.5 Net Carbs for entire recipe

1. Heat the olive oil over medium-high heat in a nonstick skillet. While the oil is heating up, beat the egg with the cream in a medium bowl. Carefully check the filets for any missed bones. When they are bone-free, dredge the filets in the egg wash and dredge in Fry Coating.

2. When the oil just begins to smoke, place the fish in the pan (this will be about 365 degrees, the perfect frying temperature).

3. Turn the fish once during the cooking process when the edges turn a golden brown. Cook the second side until brown, then drain on a paper towel and season with salt and pepper. If you're cooking a large amount of fish, preheat the oven to 275 degrees and keep the cooked filets warm on a cookie sheet until you're ready to serve.

4. Use a nice crisp cabbage leaf as a "bowl" for the coleslaw, top with a sliced dill pickle, and garnish with slices of tomato.

TIP—You can substitute a pounded chicken breast for the fish filet for a change.

Wasabi Coleslaw

Serves 8

Ingredients
1½ cups shredded green cabbage (4.5 net carbs)
1 cup shredded purple cabbage (3 net carbs)
½ cup finely julienned jicama (2.5 net carbs)
Salt and pepper
3 tablespoons Kraft Green Goddess Dressing (3 net carbs)
1 tablespoon wasabi mustard (mixed from powder or paste)
1 tablespoon sour cream (.5 net carbs)
1 tablespoon mayonnaise
1 teaspoon stevia

1.5 Net Carbs per ½ cup serving

Place the vegetables in a mixing bowl, then salt and pepper to taste. In a separate bowl, mix the green goddess dressing, wasabi, sour cream, and mayonnaise. Sweeten to your desired taste with stevia. Add the dressing to the vegetables and mix well, let stand 30 minutes, then serve.

Fry Coating

You can mix a large quantity of this coating and store it in an air-tight container in the cupboard for quick, easy meals. Use for any deep-fried foods.

Ingredients
1 bag unsweetened fried pork rinds
1 tablespoon soy flour (1 net carb)

1 Net Carb for entire recipe

Grind the pork rinds in a food processer as finely as possible, then add the soy flour. Mix the pork rinds and soy flour until well incorporated.

TIP—You can use hot and spicy or BBQ flavored pork rinds as long as no sugar has been added. Portion out only enough Fry Coating for the meal so you don't contaminate the entire batch with raw meat. If you choose to add more soy flour to the mix, be sure to add 1 net carb per tablespoon to the total carb count.

Grilled London Broil with Stir-Fry

The trick to grilling a good steak is to make sure the cooking surface is clean and hot before grilling. This ensures you'll sear in the juices. Refer to the grilling chart for beef on page 300 for cooking times and tips. I find rare meat to be the most flavorful and the most tender.

A meat thermometer is the best way to determine doneness. The temperature should read 140 degrees for rare; 160 degrees for medium, or 180 degrees for well done. Always remove the meat from the heat 5 degrees before desired cooking temperature is reached. Let the meat rest for 15 minutes prior to slicing. During this time the internal temperature of the meat will rise an additional 5 degrees.

Slicing London broil also requires a little knowledge. If you slice it properly, it will be tender; improperly, you'll be chewing shoe leather. The trick is to slice the steak against the grain. To understand this, simply picture a handful of toothpicks laid side by side on the cutting board. If you took a knife and sliced across all of the toothpicks you would be cutting across the grain. If you ran a knife lengthwise down the side of one toothpick you would be slicing with the grain. Look at the steak carefully, find the direction the grain is running, and slice across the grain.

Ingredients
1–2 pounds London broil
2 tablespoons Montreal steak seasoning
1 teaspoon olive oil
1 teaspoon sesame oil
1 teaspoon butter
1 teaspoon minced garlic (.5 net carb)
1 teaspoon minced fresh ginger
½ cup sliced red bell pepper (3 net carbs)
½ cup sliced yellow bell pepper (3 net carbs)
½ cup shredded cabbage (1.5 net carbs)
¼ cup chopped bok choy
Salt and pepper

8 Net Carbs for entire recipe

1. Preheat the grill to medium-high to high heat. Clean the grill well with a wire brush to avoid sticking.

2. Season the steak with the Montreal steak seasoning on each side.

3. When the grill reaches high heat, place the steak on the grate and close the lid for the first 5 minutes of cooking. Turn, and continue cooking until the internal temperature is 5 degrees short of your desired doneness. Remove from the heat and let rest for 15 minutes.

4. During the steak's resting period, stir-fry the veggies: In a large skillet or wok, heat the olive oil, sesame oil, and butter over medium-high heat. Start by quickly stir-frying the garlic and ginger, then toss in the peppers, cabbage, and bok choy. Stir-fry until the veggies are limp, season with salt and pepper, and remove to a plate.

5. When the meat is cooked and fully rested, cut up the steak. Add additional salt and pepper to taste, and toss with the beef. Serve, along with the veggies.

 TIP—Use leftover steak for steak and eggs the next morning.

Grilled Salmon with Zucchini, Garlic Caulimash, and Italian Green Beans

Serves 2

Buy a nice, thick salmon filet from your grocer or fishmonger. It should be large enough to feed two people. With side dishes, 5 to 6 ounces for each person is sufficient.

Ingredients
10–12 ounces 1 inch thick salmon filet
1 small zucchini, quartered lengthwise (3 net carbs)
2 tablespoons olive oil
Lemon pepper
Coarse salt
1 cup Caulimash, recipe on page 197 (3 net carbs)
1 cup green beans (6 net carbs)
1 teaspoon butter
1 tablespoon grated Romano cheese
2 fresh lemon wedges (1 net carb)

15 Net Carbs for entire recipe

1. Brush both sides of the fish and all sides of the zucchini with olive oil. Season all surfaces well with lemon pepper and coarse salt, then set aside.

2. Prepare the Caulimash as directed, using the garlic method described in the Tip section.

3. Snap the green beans and peel the strings off, then steam until tender.

4. Melt a pat of butter with 1 tablespoon olive oil in a skillet over medium-high heat. Toss the green beans in the hot skillet with salt and pepper to taste and the Romano cheese. Remove from the heat and set aside.

5. Preheat the grill to medium-high heat and clean with a wire brush. When the grill is hot, place the fish and zucchini on the grate and close the lid. Wait 5 minutes, then check the progress. When the fish and zucchini are well seared on the cooking side, flip to cook the other side. Close the lid and continue cooking for an additional 7 to 9 minutes, or until the fish is flakey.

6. Serve the fish and salmon with Caulimash and green beans. Garnish with a wedge or two of fresh lemon.

Baked Salmon and Salad

Serves 2

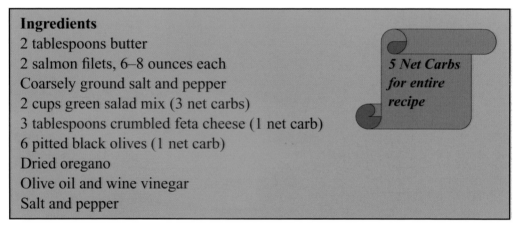

Ingredients
2 tablespoons butter
2 salmon filets, 6–8 ounces each
Coarsely ground salt and pepper
2 cups green salad mix (3 net carbs)
3 tablespoons crumbled feta cheese (1 net carb)
6 pitted black olives (1 net carb)
Dried oregano
Olive oil and wine vinegar
Salt and pepper

5 Net Carbs for entire recipe

1. Baked fish is easy and delicious. Start by preheating the oven to 375 degrees with a rack in the center. Line a cookie sheet with foil.

2. Melt the butter in the microwave and use half of it to coat the flesh side of the salmon. Place the fish, flesh side up, on the foil and season well with salt and pepper to taste. Place in the hot oven and bake for about 20 minutes (when the fish is flakey, it's done). Remove it from the oven and slip a spatula between the skin and the flesh. The fish should release from the skin very easily.

3. While the fish is baking, arrange the salad greens in 2 salad bowls. Spread half the feta cheese across the top of each salad, along with 3 olives each, and a sprinkling of oregano. Dress the salads with the oil and vinegar.

4. Serve the fish with the salads.

Italian Pork Feast with Noodles

Serves 4

Ingredients
2 tablespoons olive oil
4 country-style pork ribs
Salt and pepper
4 mild or hot Italian sausages (4 net carbs)
1 tablespoon minced garlic (2 net carbs)
2 tablespoons minced onion (1 net carb)
2 cups low-sugar pasta sauce (16 net carbs)
2 packages Tofu Shirataki Fettuccini (4 net carbs)
Grated Romano cheese
Fresh basil leaves
Fresh parsley sprigs

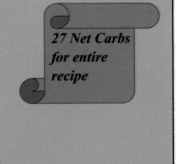

27 Net Carbs for entire recipe

1. Preheat the olive oil in a large skillet over medium heat. While the oil is heating, trim a bit of the excess pork fat from the ribs if required.

2. Salt and pepper both sides of the ribs and place in the hot skillet. Place the sausage in the skillet with the ribs and, using a spatula, move everything around for a minute or two to avoid sticking.

3. When the meat is well-browned on one side, flip the meat and cover the pan. Reduce the heat to medium-low and continue cooking for 8 to 10 minutes, checking occasionally to avoid over-browning.

4. When all sides of the meat are browned, toss in the garlic and onion, do a quick shuffle with the spatula, and reduce the heat to low. Pour in the pasta sauce and mix well, then cover and continue to cook over low heat for 30 to 45 minutes or until the pork ribs easily break apart with a fork. This meat will become very tender and succulent during the cooking process. It's important not to rush it.

5. While the meats are cooking, rinse the noodles very well, using plenty of warm water. Drain and pat the noodles dry so you don't water down the sauce, then set aside.

6. When the meat is cooked, remove it from the skillet, leaving as much sauce as possible in the pan. Raise the heat to medium and toss in the noodles. The pasta is already cooked, so you just need to heat it through. About 5 or 6 minutes should do the trick.

7. Arrange the noodles in the center of a serving dish, surrounded by the meats. Garnish with a good grinding of Romano cheese, and the fresh basil and parsley. Salt and pepper to taste and serve.

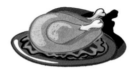

Baked Chicken and Onions

Ingredients
2 tablespoons olive oil
1 whole chicken, 4–5 pounds
2 large yellow onions, unpeeled (20 net carbs)
1 tablespoon seasoned salt
½ cup julienned red bell pepper (3 net carbs)
1 small zucchini, julienned (3 net carbs)
Salt and pepper

26 Net Carbs for entire recipe

1. Preheat the oven to 350 degrees.

2. Pour a tablespoon of olive oil into the palm of your hand and give the bird a good rubdown. Repeat the same process on the onions. Sprinkle the bird and onions with a good coating of seasoned salt and place them in an open baking dish or roasting pan. Reference the poultry roasting chart in the appendix (page 310) for cooking times. Be sure to wash your hands well after touching the raw chicken.

3. While the chicken is roasting, julienne the bell pepper and zucchini.

4. When the chicken is cooked, place it on a serving platter. Quarter the onions lengthwise and arrange the julienned veggies as a raw garnish. Salt

and pepper everything to taste. If you prefer cooked veggies to raw veggies, simply sauté them quickly in butter before serving.

TIP—If you have leftover veggies from this meal, chop them up and mix with twice as much chopped chicken meat. Add enough mayonnaise to moisten the mixture to your liking and refrigerate. Use this chicken salad as a topping on greens for a quick, easy lunch.

DESERTS

One-Minute Chocolate Cake

Ingredients
1 large egg (1 net carb)
5 teaspoons xylitol or 10 packets stevia
2 tablespoons unsweetened cocoa powder
1 tablespoon heavy cream
1 tablespoon butter, softened
1 teaspoon baking powder
½ teaspoon vanilla extract
Nonstick cooking spray
2 tablespoons Reddi-wip topping (1 net carb)

2 Net Carbs for entire recipe

1. Beat the egg with a fork in a small bowl. Add the xylitol or stevia, cocoa powder, cream, butter, baking powder, and vanilla and mix well.

2. Lightly coat an 8-ounce microwavable coffee mug with nonstick cooking spray. Pour the batter into the mug and microwave on high for 1 minute.

3. Remove the cake from the microwave and top with Reddi-wip topping. Eat the cake right from the mug.

Chocolate Chip Strawberry Shortcake

Oh, yeah! Chocolate chip strawberry shortcake! Does it get any better than this? ☺ I grew up with strawberry shortcake and I never dreamed I could eat it and still lose weight. The part of the traditional dessert that packs on the pounds is the flour and sugar in the shortcake. By replacing the shortcake with a TastyKake (available at **www.tastykake.com/products/betterforyou**) you eliminate most of the sugar from this dessert.

Ingredients
½ cup chopped strawberries (2 net carbs)
1 packet stevia or xylitol

4 tablespoons whipped cream (2 net carbs)
1 TastyKake Sensables Chocolate Chip Finger Cake
  (4 net carbs)

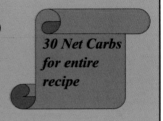

8 Net Carbs for entire recipe

1. Clean, trim, and quarter the strawberries into a small bowl. Stir in the stevia or xylitol and set aside for 15 minutes.

2. Cover the bottom of a dessert dish with whipped cream. Make your life easy and squirt it from a Reddi-wip can. ☺

3. Cut the cake into quarters and nestle the quarters into a dessert dish. Fill the dish with the strawberries and top with more Reddi-wip. Serve immediately.

Coconut Macaroons

Ingredients
3½ cups unsweetened shredded coconut (28 net carbs)
¾ cup xylitol
4 egg whites (2 net carbs)
1 teaspoon vanilla extract
½ teaspoon salt

30 Net Carbs for entire recipe

1. Preheat the oven to 300 degrees. Line a cookie sheet with parchment paper.

2. Using a double boiler, bring 2 to 3 inches of water to a boil over high heat, then reduce to a simmer.

3. Combine all the ingredients and place the mix into the top pot of your double boiler, stirring occasionally to prevent the bottom from burning. Cook until the mixture is hot and has thickened slightly, about 10 minutes.

4. With a medium cookie scoop, drop the batter onto the cookie sheet. Bake for 15–20 minutes, or until the edges of the cookies are dark golden brown.

5. Remove from the oven and let cool on the counter; the cookies will firm up as they cool. When they reach room temperature, place them in the fridge to continue firming up. Store in the refrigerator.

Crunchy Cocoa Nuts

Ingredients
Nonstick cooking spray
1 egg white (1 net carb)
¼ cup xylitol
1 teaspoon unsweetened cocoa powder
⅛ teaspoon vanilla extract
Salt
1 cup mixed unsalted walnuts, almonds, and pecans (10 net carbs)

11 Net Carbs for entire recipe

1. Preheat the oven to 325 degrees. Line a cookie sheet with foil and spray with nonstick cooking spray.

2. In a mixing bowl, whisk the egg until frothy. Whisk in the xylitol, cocoa, vanilla, and a pinch of salt. Add the nuts and stir to coat with the egg mixture.

3. Spread the nut mixture on the cookie sheet. Bake for 15–20 minutes, or until the coating has set and becomes crisp. It will cook as one flat piece, resembling brittle.

4. Cool, then break up the nuts into smaller pieces.

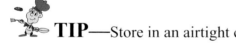 **TIP**—Store in an airtight container at room temperature.

Baked Brie on Apple Slices

Serves 4

This is one of the few times I'll use apples in a recipe due to higher carb counts. However, you can control the portions very easily by slicing the apple paper-thin. Choose a nice crisp apple like a Rome, Macintosh, or Granny Smith.

Ingredients
1 4-ounce wheel Brie cheese
1 teaspoon butter
1 apple, thinly sliced (16 net carbs)

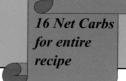

16 Net Carbs for entire recipe

1. Preheat the oven to 350 degrees.

2. Cut a big "X" in the top of the brie and place the wheel into a buttered baking dish. Bake until brown and bubbly, about 6 minutes.

3. Serve on a dinner plate surrounded by the apple slices. Limit yourself to ¼ apple (4 carbs) per serving.

Beanit Butter Cups

Makes 24 cups

Carb Not Beanit Butter is a spread made from roasted soybeans that can be used in place of peanut butter. It is available from **www.dixiediner.com**.

Ingredients
4 squares unsweetened Luker baking chocolate
¾ cup xylitol
½ cup heavy whipping cream, at room temperature
½ cup Carb Not Beanit Butter
¼ cup peanuts (7 net carbs)

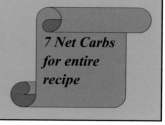

7 Net Carbs for entire recipe

1. Line a mini-muffin pan with mini-muffin liners.

2. Melt the chocolate in a double boiler. Add the xylitol to the melted chocolate and mix well. Add the cream and mix well.

3. Fill the liners one third full with the chocolate mixture. Add 1 teaspoon Beanit Butter to each one. Top with more of the chocolate mixture and drop a few peanuts on top of each cup.

4. Refrigerate for 2 hours, or until firm, and serve.

TIP—There are different brands of baking chocolate on the market but Luker brand is carb-free, making these cups a 0-carb treat! Store in the refrigerator for best results.

Beanit Butter Walnut Cookies

Ingredients
1 15-ounce jar Carb Not Beanit Butter
2 large eggs (2 net carbs)
½ cup finely chopped walnuts (4 net carbs)
¼ cup Log Cabin Sugar-Free Syrup

6 Net Carbs for entire recipe

1. Preheat the oven to 400 degrees.

2. Using an electric mixer, beat the Beanit Butter, the eggs, ¼ cup of the walnuts, and the syrup until well mixed. Roll the dough between your palms into 1-inch balls.

3. Place the remaining ¼ cup walnuts on a plate and roll the balls in the walnut pieces to coat all sides, then place on a cookie sheet. Flatten the cookies with a fork to about ¼ inch thick. Bake for 12 minutes.

4. Remove the cookies from the oven and let cool. They will be crumbly when they first come out of the oven. Refrigerate or store in the freezer to firm them up.

TIP—This is not a very sweet cookie as there is only a minuscule carb count per cookie from the walnuts. They are wonderful with coffee, and they are best eaten directly from the freezer.

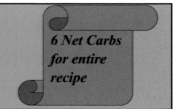

Video-supported recipe! Go to this Web site to watch me make it for you: **www.FATtoSKINNY.com/recipes.htm**.

Berry Berry Jell-O with Reddi-wip Topping

Ingredients
1 box raspberry sugar-free Jell-O
¼ cup strawberries (1 net carb)
¼ cup raspberries (2 net carbs)
¼ cup blackberries (2 net carbs)
Reddi-wip topping (add 1 net carb per 2 tablespoons)

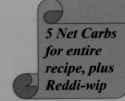

5 Net Carbs for entire recipe, plus Reddi-wip

1. Make the Jell-O following the instructions on the box, replacing the cold water with ice for a faster set. Place it in the fridge.

2. Clean and chop a few strawberries. Combine with the raspberries and blackberries and refrigerate. When the Jell-O starts to thicken, but before it sets completely, mix in the berries. Let it come to full set.

3. Serve with Reddi-wip topping.

Ice Cream Cake

Serves 4

TastyKakes Sensables are available at **www.tastykake.com/products/betterforyou**.

Ingredients
4 TastyKake Sensables Chocolate Chocolate Chip
  Finger Cakes (8 net carbs)
1 cup Breyers CarbSmart low-carb vanilla ice
  cream, softened until spreadable (8 net carbs)
½ cup Reddi-wip topping (4 net carbs)

5 Net Carbs per serving

1. Cut each cake in half lengthwise and place one half as the first layer in a dessert dish.

2. Spread a layer of low-carb ice cream onto the cakes and then top with the remaining cake.

3. Top each portion with Reddi-wip and serve.

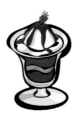

Strawberry Chocolate Ice Cream Sundae

You've got to be kidding! Ice cream sundaes on a weight loss plan? You BET, and they are wonderful.

Ingredients
¼ cup strawberries (1 net carb)
½ cup Breyers CarbSmart low-carb vanilla ice
  cream (4 net carbs)
Walden Farms Chocolate Syrup
2 tablespoons Reddi-wip topping (1 net carb)

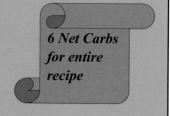

6 Net Carbs for entire recipe

Mash 2 or 3 strawberries in a bowl and quickly mix the mashed berries into the ice cream with a fork. Pour a little chocolate sauce in the bottom of a dessert dish and scoop in the ice cream. Top the ice cream with more chocolate sauce and squirt of the Reddi-wip. Top the masterpiece with a fresh berry!

Chocolate Peanut Butter Nut Fudge

Makes 38 Servings

The fudge mix and the Beanit Butter are both available from **www.dixiediner.com**.

Ingredients
1 box Dixie Diner Carb Counters Low-carb Fudge Mix (38 net carbs)
Nonstick cooking spray

1. Follow the instructions on the fudge mix package to make the fudge.

2. Coat the inside of a glass measuring cup with nonstick cooking spray. Add the baking chocolate and melt in the microwave. Stir the melted chocolate into the fudge mix. Add the Beanit Butter and nuts and mix well.

3. Add the cream, stir until the cream is incorporated, and then spread the mixture into a nonstick, 8-inch-square shallow baking pan.

4. Allow the fudge to rest on the counter for 30 minutes. Refrigerate for 2 hours before serving.

TIP—You can use peanuts or walnuts to replace the macadamia nuts. You can also use Smuckers Natural Crunchy or Smooth Peanut Butter to replace the Beanit Butter; however, the fudge will have a higher carb count.

Chocolate-Dipped Strawberries

Ingredients
¼ cup melted sugar-free chocolates
1 cup whole strawberries (4 net carbs)

4 Net Carbs for entire recipe

Melt the SUGAR-free chocolate in a double boiler until creamy. Individually dip each strawberry into the chocolate three-quarters of the way up the berry, then set on wax paper to cool.

TIP—Use cold berries to decrease the chocolate set time. Make extra—they refrigerate well.

Mango-Peach Jell-O

Ingredients
1 box peach sugar-free Jell-O
1 cup Minute Maid Light Mango–Passion Fruit juice (3 net carbs)
2 tablespoons Reddi-wip topping (1 net carb)

1 Net Carb per serving

Make the Jell-O following the instructions on the box, replacing the added cold water with juice. Refrigerate to set. Serve with Reddi-wip topping.

Strawberry Cream Cheese Crepes

Makes 4 8-inch crepes

Crepes are very easy to make. They are simply very thin pancakes used to roll up a variety of ingredients.

Ingredients
2 tablespoons New Hope Mills Pancake and Waffle Mix (1.5 net carbs)
2 large eggs (2 net carbs)
2 teaspoons water
1 tablespoon butter, plus additional for pan
4 ounces cream cheese (4 net carbs)
½ cup fresh mashed strawberries (2 net carbs)
2 whole strawberries, quartered (.5 net carb)
Reddi-wip topping (add 1 net carb per 2 tablespoons to total carb count)

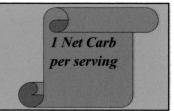

10 Net Carbs for entire recipe without Reddi-wip

1. Beat together well the New Hope Mills Pancake and Waffle Mix, eggs, and water.

2. Preheat an 8-inch nonstick skillet over medium heat. Using a stick of butter, make sure the bottom of the pan and an inch or two up the sides are greased.

3. Pour in a small amount of the batter and, using the pan's handle, lift and swirl the pan to spread the batter out thinly across the entire bottom of the pan. Cover the pan for 60 seconds. The crepe should be set on top and can now be gently removed from the pan onto a plate. Repeat the process, stacking the crepes on top of one another and separated with paper towels until you have made all the crepes you need.

4. In a mixing bowl, beat the cream cheese together with the mashed berries until well incorporated. Do not "overwork" the mixture.

5. Place a quarter of the filling into each crepe, reserving about a tablespoon of filling. Gently roll up each crepe and arrange neatly on a serving plate.

6. Top each crepe in 2 places with a small amount of the filling and "glue" the quartered strawberries to the top. Grab the Reddi-wip can, decorate the plate, and serve.

TIP—Blackberries or raspberries can be substituted, at 4 net carbs per ½ cup.

Blackberry Sorbet

Ingredients
2 tablespoons blackberries (1 net carb)
½ cup Breyers CarbSmart low-carb vanilla ice
    cream (4 net carbs)
1 tablespoons Reddi-wip topping (1 net carb)

6 Net Carbs for entire recipe

Mash the blackberries with a fork. Work the berries into the ice cream until fully incorporated and smooth. Top with Reddi-wip topping and a whole berry.

TIP—Strawberries or raspberries can be substituted. Strawberries have half the amount of carbs as blackberries; raspberries have the same carb count as blackberries.

Berry Berry Berry Applesauce Cake

This cake is so good, you'll feel like you're cheating! Made with Dixie Diners Applesauce Snackin' Cake Mix (available from **www.dixiediner.com**), it's sure to please the whole family.

Ingredients
1 package Dixie Diners Applesauce Low-Carb
  Snackin' Cake Mix (18 net carbs)
¼ cup strawberries (1 net carb)
2 tablespoons blueberries (2.5 net carbs)
¼ cup blackberries (2 net carbs)

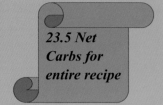
23.5 Net Carbs for entire recipe

1. Make the cake following the instructions on the package and let cool. Frost the cake, using the frosting pack supplied with the mix, and refrigerate.

2. Clean and trim the berries, then pat them dry and refrigerate. Once everything is cold, arrange the berries in any design you would like and serve!

TIP—Make sure to keep the cake cold until serving time.

Strawberry Mousse

2 Net Carbs for entire recipe

Ingredients
½ cup strawberries (2 net carbs)
1 box strawberry sugar-free Jell-O
½ cup heavy whipping cream

1. Chop some strawberries into small ¼-inch pieces and refrigerate (it's

very important to make them cold before using them in this recipe).

2. Make the Jell-O following the instructions on the box and place it in the fridge to begin setting. It's a good idea to use ice-cold water to speed up the time in which the Jell-O begins to set. You can even use ice-cold Diet Rite Black Cherry Soda in place of the water if you wish.

3. You're not going to allow the Jell-O to set completely before finishing this recipe; you're going to keep an eye on it and pull it out of the fridge when it starts getting really thick, but not yet set. You're looking for the consistency of thick pancake batter. Timeframes differ depending on your climate, but 45 minutes is about right for me.

4. The next task is to make whipped cream. If you've never made home-made whipped cream before, don't worry—it's easy. All you need is a stand mixer or a hand mixer, a heavy whipping cream, and a cold bowl. I like to use a metal bowl that I've put in the fridge for about an hour, and a hand mixer. You want to make an equal quantity of whipped cream to the quantity of finished Jell-O, so if you make 1 box of Jell-O, which yields 2 cups, you'll need 2 cups whipped cream. If you make 2 boxes of Jell-O, you'll need 4 cups whipped cream, and so on. Use ½ cup cream for each box of Jell-O used to yield 2 cups whipped cream. Whip the heavy cream in a cold metal bowl until it's stiff. You'll know it's right when you pull up the mixer beaters and stiff peaks stand straight up. If the Jell-O has now thickened to the proper consistency, then proceed to the next step. If not, put the whipped cream in the fridge and be patient. ☺

5. Once the Jell-O has thickened, slowly add it to the finished whipped cream and gently fold together. Add the chopped strawberries into the mix-ture and once again gently fold in.

6. Now you have a choice to make: do you want the desserts to set inside individual dessert dishes, or do you want to spoon out servings from a larger bowl? I use a Tupperware container large enough to hold the entire recipe and I scoop out servings into individual serving dishes. That way I get the "fluffy" look on top. Whichever you choose, transfer the mixture into the

container(s) and place in the fridge to fully set. In a few hours you will have a delicious sugar-free dessert that will rival any you've tasted in the past.

TIP—You can substitute blackberries or raspberries for the strawberries or you can have a mixture of berries (double the berry carb count if using blackberries or raspberries). Use a different flavor of sugar-free Jell-O, such as strawberry-banana or mixed fruit, if you wish.

Video-supported recipe! Go to this Web site to watch me make it for you: **www.FATtoSKINNY.com/recipes.htm**.

Chocolate Mousse

Try this rich mousse with House Foods silken tofu, available at **www.house-foods.com**.

Ingredients
1 14-ounce package House Foods silken tofu (6 net carbs)
¼ cup xylitol
1½ tablespoons unsweetened cocoa powder (1.5 net carbs)
Reddi-wip topping (add 1 net carb per 2 tablespoons to carb total)
¼ cup raspberries (2 net carbs)
4 fresh mint leaves

9.5 Net Carbs for entire recipe without Reddi-wip

Combine the tofu, xylitol, and cocoa powder in a food processor, blending until extra creamy and whipped. Serve in delightful crystal martini glasses, each topped with a dollop of Reddi-wip. Garnish with raspberries and mint.

TIP—Switch it up a bit by adding a teaspoon of peppermint extract to the food processor to make chocolate-mint mousse. Or add a tablespoon of extra creamy peanut butter for a new take on an old favorite.

Double Chocolate Raspberry Sundae

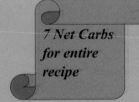

Ingredients
2 tablespoons Reddi-wip topping (1 net carb)
2 tablespoons raspberries (1 net carb)
½ cup Breyers CarbSmart Chocolate Ice Cream
  (4 net carbs)
2 tablespoons Chocolate Reddi-wip topping (1 net carb)

7 Net Carbs for entire recipe

1. Start with a frozen dessert dish. Squirt a good shot of regular, white Reddi-wip in the bottom of the dish and throw in a couple raspberries. Follow with a scoop of the ice cream.

2. Squirt in another good shot of white Reddi-wip, add a couple more raspberries and follow with another scoop of chocolate ice cream. Top with a small mountain of chocolate Reddi-wip topping and the remaining raspberries.

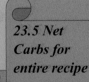 **TIP**—Stick to the serving size on the ice cream and splurge on the berries and whipped cream. Substitute strawberries or blackberries for a different variation.

Key Lime Pie

Ingredients
Almond Meal Pie Crust, recipe on page 277 (7 net carbs)
Sweetened Condensed Milk, recipe on page 277 (3.5 net
  carbs)
½ cup sour cream (4 net carbs)
½ cup key lime juice (8 net carbs)
1 tablespoon grated lime zest (1 net carb)
Whipped cream, optional

23.5 Net Carbs for entire recipe

1. Preheat the oven to 325 degrees.

2. Prepare the Almond Meal Pie Crust and Sweetened Condensed Milk.

3. In a medium bowl, combine the Sweetened Condensed Milk, sour cream, lime juice, and lime zest. Mix well and pour into the pie crust.

4. Bake for 8 to 12 minutes, until tiny pinhole bubbles burst on the surface of the pie. Do not allow the top of the pie to brown.

5. Chill the pie thoroughly before serving. Garnish with whipped cream if desired.

TIP—You can switch this up and make a lemon pie by replacing the key lime juice with lemon juice and the lime zest with lemon zest.

Pumpkin Tofu Cheesecake

Ingredients
Nut Crust, optional, recipe on page 276 (14 net carbs)
1½ pounds silken tofu (9 net carbs)
1 15-ounce can pumpkin puree (15 net carbs)
12 ounces cream cheese (12 net carbs)
¼ cup xylitol
1 teaspoon cinnamon
1 tablespoon vanilla extract
½ teaspoon ground nutmeg
Reddi-wip topping (add 1 net carb per 2 tablespoons to total carb count)

36 Net Carbs for entire recipe without crust

1. Preheat the oven to 350 degrees. Bring all the ingredients to room temperature. If you want a crust, make the Nut Crust now.

2. In a food processor or blender, puree the tofu until smooth, then add in all the other ingredients except whipped cream. Scrape the sides of the bowl until well mixed.

3. If you've prepared a crust, pour the mixture into it. If you're going crust-free, butter a springform pan well and pour in the mixture. Bake for an hour, until the center is firm (it may require more time depending on altitude and oven).

4. Turn the oven off and leave the cheesecake in the oven for 1 more hour.

5. Remove the cheesecake from the oven and let it cool to room temperature. Place in the fridge overnight.

6. Serve with Reddi-wip topping.

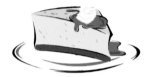

Strawberry Cottage Cheesecake

Ingredients
Nut Crust, recipe on page 276 (14 net carbs)
3 boxes sugar-free strawberry Jell-O
12 ounces cottage cheese (9 net carbs)
3 cups cold strawberries, trimmed and sliced (12 net carbs)
Reddi-wip topping (add 1 net carb per 2 tablespoons to total carb count)

35 Net Carbs for entire recipe without Reddi-wip

1. Prepare the Nut Crust. Cool the crust to room temperature, then place the pan in the freezer.

2. Dissolve the powder from 2 boxes of Jell-O in 1 cup hot water. Stir in 1 cup cold water. Combine the mixture with the cottage cheese in a food processor and blend well.

3. Pour the mixture on top of the frozen crust and refrigerate until firm.

4. When the cheesecake is firm, place 2 cups of the strawberries on top of the set Jell-O.

5. Prepare the remaining box of gelatin following the package instructions. Use ice water for the second cup of water. Gently pour the liquid on top of the strawberries. Put the cheesecake back in fridge until set.

6. Top the cheesecake with Reddi-wip and the remaining strawberries.

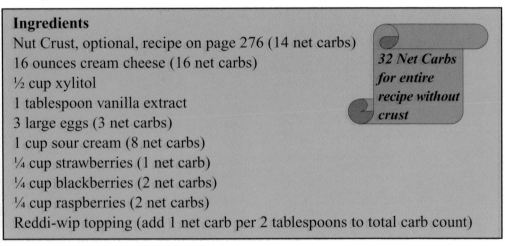 **TIP**—This recipe can be made crust-free, saving 14 net carbs, using a deep-dish pie pan or a frozen springform pan. Many springform cheesecake pans will leak if the filling is very thin. This filling will be thin at the beginning of the process, so if you wish to use a springform pan to have a crust-free cake, freeze the pan prior to use. This trick usually forces the gelatin to coagulate quickly, resolving the leak issue. If you decide not to go crust-free, freezing the crust protects it from becoming soggy.

Berry, Berrylicious Cheesecake

This pie is crust-free, but you may add a crust if you like.

Ingredients
Nut Crust, optional, recipe on page 276 (14 net carbs)
16 ounces cream cheese (16 net carbs)
½ cup xylitol
1 tablespoon vanilla extract
3 large eggs (3 net carbs)
1 cup sour cream (8 net carbs)
¼ cup strawberries (1 net carb)
¼ cup blackberries (2 net carbs)
¼ cup raspberries (2 net carbs)
Reddi-wip topping (add 1 net carb per 2 tablespoons to total carb count)

32 Net Carbs for entire recipe without crust

1. Preheat the oven to 350 degrees.

2. If using a crust, prepare the Nut Crust and cool.

3. Beat the cream cheese, xylitol, and vanilla in a mixing bowl until well

blended. Beat in the eggs on low speed, one at a time. Gently fold in the sour cream.

4. If you've prepared a crust, pour the mixture on top of it. If you're going crust-free, butter a springform pan well and pour the mixture into it.

5. Bake for 1 hour until firm. Turn off the heat and leave the cheesecake in the oven for 1 hour.

6. Cool to room temperature, then refrigerate overnight.

7. Top with berries and Reddi-wip, and serve.

No-Bake Cheesecake

Ingredients
2 envelopes Knox unflavored gelatin
½ cup plus 2 tablespoons xylitol
16 ounces cream cheese (16 net carbs)
2 teaspoons vanilla
1 cup strawberries, trimmed and chopped (4 net carbs)
¼ cup water

20 Net Carbs for entire recipe

1. Mix the gelatin powder and ½ cup xylitol in a bowl. Add 2 cups boiling water and stir until the powder is completely dissolved.

2. Beat the cream cheese and vanilla together in a mixing bowl until smooth and creamy. Slowly beat in the gelatin-xylitol mixture until well combined.

3. Pour the mixture into a deep-dish pie pan and refrigerate for 3 hours.

4. Put the strawberries in a saucepan on the stove. Add ¼ cup water and the remaining 2 tablespoons xylitol and mix well. Stirring continuously to avoid sticking, cook the strawberries over medium heat for about 7 to 9 minutes, or until thick. Cool completely and pour over the cheesecake. Slice and serve.

GG Bran Sprinkles Cheesecake Crust

GG Bran Sprinkles are available at **www.brancrispbread.com**.

Ingredients
⅓ cup GG Bran Sprinkles (4 net carbs)
1 large egg, beaten (1 net carb)
3 packets stevia
1 teaspoon butter to grease cheesecake pan

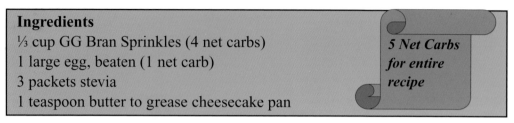

5 Net Carbs for entire recipe

Preheat the oven to 350 degrees. Mix the GG Bran Sprinkles with the egg and stevia. Press the mixture into a well-greased cheesecake pan and bake for 10 to 15 minutes. Remove from the oven and cool.

Nut Crust

Ingredients
1½ cups ground walnuts, almonds, or hazelnuts
  (13 net carbs)
1 large egg (1 net carb)
⅛ cup xylitol or 2 packets stevia
1 teaspoon butter to grease cheesecake pan

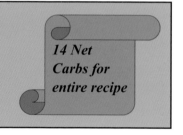

14 Net Carbs for entire recipe

1. Preheat the oven to 350 degrees. Grease a springform pan.

2. Finely chop the nuts in a food processor. Add the egg and xylitol or stevia to the processor and process until well blended. Press the dough into the bottom of the pan.

3. Bake the crust for 10 to 12 minutes. Remove from the oven and cool.

Almond Meal Pie Crust

Ingredients
1½ cups unblanched almond meal (6 net carbs)
3 tablespoons melted butter
3 tablespoons xylitol
1 large egg, lightly beaten (1 net carb)
1 teaspoon butter to grease pan

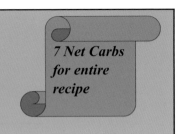

7 Net Carbs for entire recipe

1. Preheat the oven to 350 degrees.

2. In a small mixing bowl, combine the almond meal, butter, and xylitol. Mix with a fork, then add the egg and continue mixing until well incorporated.

3. Press the dough into a 9-inch greased pie pan with your fingertips or a spoon.

4. Bake for 10 to 12 minutes, until the crust is begins to brown. After 8 minutes, check every minute or so, because once it starts to brown it goes quickly.

5. Remove from the oven and cool.

Sweetened Condensed Milk

Ingredients
2½ cups heavy cream
6 egg yolks (3.5 net carbs)
6 tablespoons xylitol
1 teaspoon vanilla extract

3.5 Net Carbs for entire recipe

Whisk together the heavy cream, egg yolks, xylitol, and vanilla in a saucepan. Cook over low heat, stirring until thick. Cool completely and store in a non-metallic covered container in the fridge.

Easy Custard

Ingredients
2 cups whipping cream
2 large eggs (2 net carbs)
2 tablespoons xylitol
⅛ teaspoon salt
Ground nutmeg

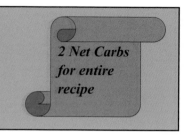

2 Net Carbs for entire recipe

1. Preheat the oven to 325 degrees.

2. Beat together the cream, eggs, xylitol, and salt.

3. Pour the mixture into custard cups so that they're 80 percent full, then sprinkle with nutmeg. Place the cups in a baking dish and place the baking dish into the oven. Carefully pour hot water into the baking dish up to the fill-line on the custard cups.

4. Bake for 40 to 45 minutes, until the custard is set (a knife inserted in the center should come out clean).

Brownies

Ingredients
½ cup butter or margarine, melted
½ cup unsweetened cocoa
¾ cup xylitol
2 large eggs (2 net carbs)
¼ cup heavy cream
1 teaspoon vanilla
½ cup unblanched almond meal (2 net carbs)
3 tablespoons soy flour (3 net carbs)
½ teaspoon baking powder
¼ teaspoon salt

7 Net Carbs for entire recipe

1. Preheat the oven to 350 degrees. Grease a 9-inch square pan.

2. Stir together the butter and cocoa in a mixing bowl. Add the xylitol, eggs, cream, and vanilla and beat until smooth. Add the almond meal, soy flour, baking powder, and salt. Mix to combine.

3. Spread the batter into the baking pan and bake about 20 minutes, or until a wooden toothpick inserted into the center comes out clean.

4. Let cool completely before cutting into squares and serving.

TIP—Use NOW brand unblanched almond meal. It has the lowest carb count I've found: 4 net grams per cup. I buy mine at **Amazon.com**, but many whole food stores and health food stores stock it.

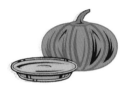

Crust-Free Pumpkin Pie

Ingredients
3 cups mashed cooked pumpkin or canned pumpkin puree (24 net carbs)
1⅓ cups heavy cream
½ cup xylitol
3 large eggs (3 net carbs)
2 teaspoons cinnamon
1 teaspoon allspice
1 teaspoon ground cloves
½ teaspoon ground ginger
Whipped cream
Freshly ground nutmeg
1 teaspoon butter to grease pan

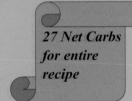

27 Net Carbs for entire recipe

1. Preheat the oven to 425 degrees.

2. Process all the ingredients in a food processor until smooth. Pour the mixture into a well-greased pie pan (I like to use glass pans).

3. Bake for 15 minutes, then reduce the heat to 350 degrees and cook another 60 minutes.

4. Cool completely before cutting; serve with whipped cream and a grinding of nutmeg on top.

Video-supported recipe! Go to this Web site to watch me make it for you: **www.FATtoSKINNY.com/recipes.htm**.

Pumpkin Cookies

Ingredients
1 cup soy flour (16 net carbs)
1 cup unblanched almond meal (4 net carbs)
½ cup soy protein powder
1 teaspoon baking powder
1 teaspoon baking soda
3 teaspoons ground cinnamon
½ teaspoon ground nutmeg
½ teaspoon ground cloves
¼ teaspoon salt
½ cup butter, softened, plus 2 teaspoons to grease cookie sheet
¾ cups xylitol
1 cup canned pumpkin puree (8 net carbs)
1 large egg (1 net carb)
2 teaspoons vanilla extract

29 Net Carbs for entire recipe

1. Preheat the oven to 350 degrees. Grease a cookie sheet with butter.

2. Combine the soy flours, almond meal, protein powder, baking powder, baking soda, cinnamon, nutmeg, cloves, and salt; set aside.

3. In a medium bowl, cream together the butter and xylitol. Add the pumpkin, egg, and 1 teaspoon vanilla and beat until creamy. Add in the dry ingredients and mix well.

4. Drop the batter by tablespoonfuls onto the cookie sheet and flatten slightly with a fork. Bake for 18 to 20 minutes, or until firm.

5. Place the cookies on a cooling rack and let cool prior to serving.

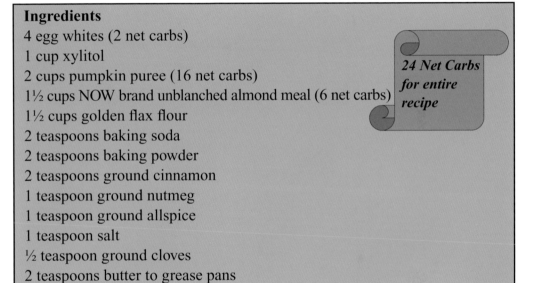

Video-supported recipe! Go to this Web site to watch me make it for you: **www.FATtoSKINNY.com/recipes.htm.**

Pumpkin Bread

Makes 2 loaves

Ingredients
4 egg whites (2 net carbs)
1 cup xylitol
2 cups pumpkin puree (16 net carbs)
1½ cups NOW brand unblanched almond meal (6 net carbs)
1½ cups golden flax flour
2 teaspoons baking soda
2 teaspoons baking powder
2 teaspoons ground cinnamon
1 teaspoon ground nutmeg
1 teaspoon ground allspice
1 teaspoon salt
½ teaspoon ground cloves
2 teaspoons butter to grease pans

24 Net Carbs for entire recipe

1. Preheat the oven to 350 degrees. Grease 2 loaf pans (or 4 small pans).

2. Beat the egg whites and xylitol together until well mixed and lightened, but not to the point of stiffness. Add the pumpkin puree (do not use pumpkin pie filling) and whisk together well.

3. In a separate bowl, mix all the dry ingredients and spices. Pour the dry ingredients into the wet ingredients and whisk well.

4. Pour the batter into the greased loaf pans. Bake for 60 minutes or until a toothpick inserted into the middle comes out clean.

5. Let cool before removing from the pans, then slice. These breads freeze well in a zippered plastic freezer bag.

TIP—Serve with spicy pumpkin butter . . . YUM! Cream together 2 tablespoons soft butter and 1 teaspoon pumpkin pie spice.

Video-supported recipe! Go to this Web site to watch me make it for you: **www.FATtoSKINNY.com/recipes.htm**.

Lemon Ice Cream

Ingredients
2 cups heavy cream
1 cup unsweetened vanilla almond milk (1 net carb)
½ cup xylitol
3 tablespoons vanilla extract
⅛ teaspoon salt
2 large eggs (2 net carbs)
3 tablespoons crushed sugar-free lemon candy
1 tablespoon lemon extract

3 Net Carbs for entire recipe

1. Combine the cream, almond milk, xylitol, vanilla, and salt in a heavy saucepan. Heat the cream mixture just to a boil.

2. Meanwhile, whisk the eggs in a large bowl. Add the hot cream mixture to the eggs in a slow stream while vigorously whisking to avoid curdling the eggs.

3. Pour the mixture back into the saucepan and cook over medium heat, stirring constantly, until slightly thickened and a thermometer reads 170 degrees.

4. Pour the custard into a bowl and cool to room temperature, stirring occasionally.

5. Cover with plastic wrap and refrigerate until cold, at least 5 hours or overnight. (The colder the mix, the better the ice cream.)

6. Remove from the fridge when cold and stir well. Pour into an ice cream maker and process following the manufacturer's instructions. Keep an eye on the ice cream as it processes. When ice cream starts to become very thick, add the lemon extract and lemon candy. For my machine this is usually occurs within the last 5 minutes of processing.

7. Serve immediately for soft-serve ice cream, or place into freezer for a firmer ice cream.

TIP—Use this custard ice cream base for different flavored ice creams by changing the extract and the candy. One of my favorites is peppermint ice cream. Replace the lemon extract and candy with peppermint extract and sugar-free crushed peppermint candy.

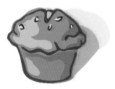

Maple Walnut Muffins

Makes 18 large muffins

Ingredients
2 cups NOW Almond Flour (8 net carbs)
1 tablespoon baking powder
½ teaspoon salt
¼ cup butter softened
¼ cup xylitol

Less than 1 net carb per muffin

2 teaspoons vanilla extract
¼ cup Log Cabin Sugar Free Syrup
2 large eggs (2 net carbs)
½ cup heavy whipping cream
½ cup chopped walnuts (4 net carbs)
1. Preheat the oven to 375 degrees. Line a muffin pan with paper baking cups.

2. Mix together the almond meal, baking powder, and salt in a medium bowl.

3. In a mixing bowl, beat the butter, xylitol, and vanilla together until light and fluffy. Stir in the syrup and eggs and beat until mixed. Add the dry ingredients alternately with the cream, and mix well. Stir in the walnuts.

4. Spoon the batter into the muffin pan, filling each cup about three-quarters full.

5. Bake for 18 to 20 minutes, or until a toothpick inserted into the center comes out clean.

6. Put the muffins on a wire rack to set and cool completely before serving. If you overcook these, they will be crumbly.

Hazelnut Soufflé

Ingredients
Nonstick cooking spray
2 tablespoons finely chopped hazelnuts (1 net carb)
⅛ cup xylitol
4 large eggs (4 net carbs)
¼ teaspoon cream of tartar
2 tablespoons hazelnut extract
Whipped cream, for serving

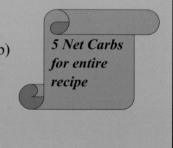

5 Net Carbs for entire recipe

1. Preheat the oven to 375 degrees. Prepare the soufflé dish: spray the dish with nonstick cooking spray and wrap it in foil so you have 4 additional inches in height. (The soufflé will rise above soufflé dish.) Set aside.

2. Mix the hazelnuts and xylitol in a small bowl and set aside.

3. Separate the eggs. Put the whites in a large mixing bowl and the yolks in a medium bowl. Beat the egg yolks and set aside.

4. Add the cream of tartar to the egg whites and, using a stand or hand mixer, beat until the eggs have formed stiff peaks. With the mixer running, slowly add the hazelnut mixture and then the hazelnut extract.

5. Scoop out about a cup of egg white–hazelnut mixture and gently mix it into the yolks to lighten them up. Very gently fold the egg yolk mixture into the egg white bowl.

6. Carefully transfer the mixture into the prepared soufflé dish.

7. Very gently place the dish into the oven and bake for 35 to 40 minutes, or until firm. Serve warm, with a dollop of whipped cream.

TIP—Soufflés are lots of fun, easy to make, and very versatile. Add Walden Farms sugar-free chocolate or caramel sauce for a nice variation.

KITCHEN SECRETS UNRAVELED

Instead of?

Many people fail on eating plans that remove their favorite foods because they hate *losing* their favorite foods. You don't have to go without; you simply need to *replace*. Use the "Instead of" list below and experience some of your favorite foods with a little different flavor.

Instead of PASTA, substitute spaghetti squash, julienned zucchini, Shirataki Tofu Pasta, or Miracle Noodles.

TIP—Miracle Noodles and Shirataki Tofu Noodles do not freeze well.

Instead of LASAGNA NOODLES, substitute thin slices of zucchini or eggplant cut lengthwise.

Instead of MASHED POTATOES, substitute cauliflower Caulimash. Steam a head of cauliflower until tender, drain very well, and pat dry with paper towels. Using a hand masher, roughly mash the cauliflower in the cooking pot with 1 tablespoon mayonnaise and 1 tablespoon butter. Salt and pepper to taste, then place the mixture into a food processor. Process until smooth, adding extra mayo if needed.

Instead of FRIED POTATOES, substitute pan-fried jicama. In a skillet, place small, diced jicama in an inch of lightly salted water. Boil the jicama uncovered until the pan is dry. Add a tablespoon of olive oil and a teaspoon of butter to the skillet, fry over medium heat for 6 to 7 minutes, and serve immediately. Jicama always retains a bit of a crunch.

Instead of BAKED POTATOES, substitute a chayote squash. Punch a couple of fork holes in the squash and microwave for 5 to 8 minutes, or until fork-tender. Serve as you would a baked potato, with sour cream and butter.

Instead of FRIED FOOD COATING, substitute unsweetened pork rinds finely ground in a food processor with a little soy flour added to lighten the mix.

Instead of CORNSTARCH GRAVY THICKENER, substitute ThickenThin or xanthan gum, available at **www.amazon. com**.

Instead of BREAD, substitute romaine lettuce leaves, GG Bran Crispbread, or low-carb tortillas.

Instead of FLOUR TORTILLAS, substitute La Tortilla Factory tortillas.

Instead of SUGAR SODA, substitute SUGAR-free soda. Get creative, try some Italian soda. Simply pick up various flavors of SUGAR-free syrups and seltzer water. Pour a shot glass of flavored syrup over ice, add a tablespoon of heavy whipping cream, and top off the glass with soda water.

Instead of SUGAR, substitute stevia or xylitol sweetener.

Instead of PIZZA, use low-carb tortillas as a base for a personal pizza loaded with cheese, meats, and veggies from the list.

Instead of RICE or COUSCOUS, process raw cauliflower in a food processer using the chopping blade. Process until the cauliflower is ground up and resembles rice. Process the cauliflower a little finer for a couscous consistency.

Your personal **"Instead of"** list will grow as you play around with your ingredients, as will your recipes. Don't be afraid to try new ideas as they present themselves to you. I look forward to reading YOUR recipes.

Send them to **dougvarrieur@FATtoSKINNY.com**.

ESCAPE FROM THE KITCHEN!

How to eat at:

RESTAURANTS

Stick to protein! Remember this rule:

Meats and Greens Will Make You Lean

Sugar and Carbs Will Make You Large

You can eat out at most restaurants simply by scoping out the sugar on the menu. Be vocal with the waitstaff. Tell them you are on a no-sugar eating plan and wish to adjust your plate. No thank you to the bread and chips. No thank you to the baked potato, rice, and carrots. Yes please to the grilled meat, fish, or chicken. Yes please to the green veggies and salads. Oh, by the way, can you make me up a bowl of fresh strawberries with whipped cream for dessert? You'll be surprised at how helpful your waitstaff will be to your needs—after all, it's their tip! ☺ Carry your copy of the **FAT TO SKINNY Sugar and Carb Counter** with you and, when in doubt, simply check the food in the book to make sure you're within guidelines.

DINNER PARTIES AND EVENTS

Eating at dinner parties and events is very simple: always bring a dish to the party. This way, you ensure that a low-sugar option will always be available for you. I find more often than not my host and hostess not only appreciate the contribution, they also appreciate my story. It never ceases to amaze me as I watch my dish disappear onto the plates of other guests. I also like to bring a dessert such as fresh berries and Reddi-wip or some low-carb ice cream. Inevitably, when I next visit my host for another dinner party, low-sugar cooking is always the fare.

THE MOVIES

Heading out to the movies after dinner? No problem! Simply make sure you have a bag of roasted almonds and some sugar-free candy with you when you go in. Sugar-free soda will be available at the theater.

HOW TO ROAST MEATS AND POULTRY

Roasting large cuts of meat and poultry is intimidating to many people. If you're one of them, don't feel bad . . . you're in good company. ☺ This chapter will make each of your experiences painless.

You remember those rules don't you? You read about them at the beginning of the recipe section.

Roasting your own meats and poultry has many benefits. You'll enjoy a wonderful meal and you'll have leftovers for snack trays and other recipes. Your trips to the deli will be dramatically reduced and your cost per pound for ham, turkey, and beef will be about 75 percent less at the register. Your meats will be fresher and they won't contain all the added salts and preservatives found in many deli meats.

Because of all these wonderful benefits, you should plan on roasting something once a week: a turkey one week, a ham the next. Up comes a big chicken or two with a roast beef tailing. Let's not forget a good pork loin and a lamb roast.

I know what you're thinking . . . "Turkey all week long, turkey this, turkey that! YUK!" Not to worry, simply slice up the bird, divide it out, and freeze it in meal-sized portions. As your weeks progresses, you soon have a variety of meats and poultry in the freezer waiting your bidding. You'll have your own deli in the kitchen. ☺

Essential tools for roasting are a nonstick roasting pan with a rack, a good spice rub, and a meat thermometer.

Next you'll need a very hot oven—450 degrees—to begin the cooking process. All roasts and poultry start the same, 450 degrees for the first 15 minutes to sear the food. The temperature is reduced after that to finish the roasting process. Always preheat your oven when possible.

Let's start with beef.

Beef

There are all sorts of beef roasts, from round to chuck and everything in between. I'm going to concentrate on the roasts you're most likely to buy.

Top Round Prime Rib

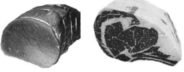

Rib Eye from which comes Rib Eye Steaks

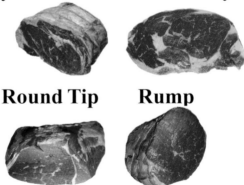

Round Tip   Rump

Top Loin from which comes New York Strips

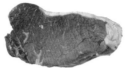

As you can see from the pictures, there is a major difference in **FAT** content in these roasts. The roast with the least "marbling," (a fancy word for **FAT** content) is the top round. The roast with the most marbling is the prime rib. Marbling makes the meat more tender simply because the **FAT** melts away during cooking, leaving gaps in the meat. The fat does double duty by basting the roast as it cooks.

If your beef roast has a layer of fat on top more than ½-inch thick (as in the photo of the prime rib), you'll want to trim off the excess fat. Simply take a sharp chef's knife and run it across the top of the roast, cutting away the excess fat but leaving ¼ to ½ inch of fat intact. This is best illustrated in the photo of the rib eye. You want to leave some because that fat will self-baste your roast. Once trimmed, generously sprinkle the roast with coarse salt and ground pepper or your favorite spice rub. Place the roast in a shallow baking pan (I like a cast iron skillet) on a rack and place it in a hot oven preheated to 450 degrees. Cook at high heat for 15 minutes, then reduce the heat to 325 degrees for the remainder of the cooking time.

I suggest you buy a good meat thermometer; they are not expensive and they will keep you out of trouble. About three-quarters of the way through the cooking time, check the meat's internal temperature by sticking the thermometer into the center of the roast, away from bone. Ovens vary in temperature, so it's a good idea to keep an eye on it.

Once the roast has reached the proper temperature, remove it from the oven and **let stand 15 to 20 minutes** prior to carving. Letting the roast stand prevents the juices from running out of the roast, which would leave it dry.

Let's discuss the roasts individually. Top round will be dry and tough if cooked anywhere above medium doneness. If you wish to cook your top round above medium, you'll need to cook it as a pot roast with plenty of liquid such as beef broth. I prefer to use cooking bags when roasting pot roasts.

Prime rib will be the most tender, the most expensive, and carry the most fat. It's a wonderful treat. Look for it on sale; I see it several times per year. When it goes on sale, pick up an extra or two for your freezer. It will stay fairly tender at all levels of doneness, but will be most tender at rare to medium-rare.

Rib eye roasts are excellent. Buy one big enough to cut off a couple of rib eye steaks for your freezer prior to roasting. It will stay fairly tender at all levels of doneness, but will be most tender at rare to medium-rare.

Eye round, round tip, and rump make the best all-around "slicing" roasts for thinly sliced beef. Cook them rare to medium-rare for the best results. Round tip and rump roasts will get tougher as they cook. If you desire well-done meat, you'll need to cook them as pot roasts with plenty of liquid such as beef broth.

Top loin roasts are also excellent. Like the rib eye, buy one big enough to cut off a couple of steaks for your freezer prior to roasting (these will be New York strip steaks). It will stay fairly tender at all levels of doneness, but will be most tender at rare to medium-rare.

Prime rib can be fairly expensive, so some advance preparation should be taken. Here are the questions that need to be answered: how big a roast, how many people are you serving, and how long do you cook it? Below, you'll find the charts I've prepared for you to answer those questions. Remember, the more well done the meat is cooked, the tougher it will be. Personally, I prefer my roast rare; it will melt in your mouth.

Different cuts of beef require different cooking methods. More tender cuts of meat return much better results when dry-roasted. For your best results, dry roast methods (on a rack in a roasting pan) should be limited to prime rib roasts, rib eye roasts, tenderloins, tri-tip roasts, sirloin roasts, and rump roasts.

That doesn't mean you can't get good cooking results with more tough and usually less expensive cuts of meat such as chuck roasts, eye of round roasts, and top round roasts. You simply employ a different cooking method, referred to as braising.

Braising is easy. In a nutshell, braising is defined as cooking at a low temperature in a pot or bag with a tight-fitting lid and a small amount of liquid. I like to make my life easy when braising roasts. I buy an oven-safe roasting bag from the market, place my seasoned roast in it, pour in ½ to ¾ cups beef broth and plop it in the oven for the prescribed time. When the roast is done, the roast and gravy are removed and the bag gets tossed . . . no fuss . . . no muss. ☺

Prime Rib Chart

Roast Size	Roast Weight in pounds	Total Cooking Time	Internal Temperature (Rare)
2 rib roast	3¾–5	55–70 minutes	120°F
3 rib roast	5¾–8	1½–1¾ hours	120°F
4 rib roast	8¾–10	1¾–2¼ hours	120°F
5 rib roast	10¾–13	2¼–2¾ hours	120°F
6 rib roast	13¾–16	3–3¼ hours	120°F
7 rib roast	16¾–19	3¼–4 hours	120°F

How Do You Like Your Meat?		
Doneness	Internal Temp	Color
Rare	120–125°F	Bright red
Medium-rare	130–135°F	Light red, with slight browning around the edges
Medium	140–145°F	Pink center, with wide brown edges
Medium-well	150–155°F	No visible pink color
Well done	160°F and above	Brown throughout

Whichever size rib you buy, a few rules pertain to all. First, make sure to bring the roast to room temperature all the way through before cooking. Simply leave your fully defrosted roast on the counter until room temperature is reached.

As mentioned, I like my prime rib rare. To carve, run a knife along the ribs first and cut them away. Then you can cut smaller slices without interference from the bones.

Fail-Proof Dry-Roast Method for Beef

Referring to the spice chart on page 314, season the roast with your preferred herbs and spices. Place the roast, fat side up, on a rack in a shallow roasting pan (a pan that is too tall will result in insufficient browning). Stick an oven-safe meat thermometer into the thickest part of the meat. Be sure to stop in the middle and to avoid the bone. Do not add water; do not cover. Roast the meat uncovered up to 5 degrees below the desired doneness, then remove from the oven. The beef will continue to cook for the next 10 to 15 minutes on your counter. This will result in the desired finished doneness. Let the roast stand 20 minutes before slicing. This allows the juices to coagulate and avoids resulting in a dry roast.

Roasting Chart for Beef

Cut	Weight in pounds	Cook Temp.	Approx. Cooking Time
Prime rib roast	4–6	325°F	26–30 minutes/pound
Prime rib roast	6–8	325°F	23–25 minutes/pound
Prime rib roast	8–10	325°F	19–21 minutes/pound
Rib eye boneless	3–4	350°F	23–30 minutes/pound
Rib eye boneless	4–6	350°F	18–20 minutes/pound
Rib eye boneless	8–10	350°F	13–15 minutes/pound
Round tip roast	2½–4	325°F	30–35 minutes/pound
Round tip roast	4–6	325°F	25–30 minutes/pound
Round tip roast	8–10	325°F	18–22 minutes/pound
Tenderloin roast	2–3	425°F	35–40 minutes total
Tenderloin roast	4–6	425°F	45–60 minutes total
Top loin	4–6	325°F	17–21 minutes/pound
Strip loin roast	6–8	325°F	14–17 minutes/pound
Top sirloin roast	2–4	350°F	16–20 minutes/pound
Top round roast	2½–4	325°F	25–30 minutes/pound
Top round roast	4–6	325°F	20–25 minutes/pound
Top round roast	6–10	325°F	17–19 minutes/pound
Tri-tip roast	1½–2	425°F	30–40 minutes total
Eye round roast	2–3	325°F	1½–1¾ hours total

Fail-Proof Braising Method for Beef

Season the roast with your preferred herbs and spices. Place the roast, fat side up, in a store-bought roasting bag or in a Dutch oven with a tight-fitting lid. Pour in ½ to ¾ cup of chicken or beef broth. If you prefer, beer, water, boxed onion soup mix (watch the label for carbs), or wine can be used instead. Bake in the roasting bag or Dutch oven for the prescribed time (see the following chart).

Braising Chart for Beef

CUT	THICKNESS/ WEIGHT	TOTAL COOKING TIME
Shoulder roast	1–1½ inches	1¾–2¼ hours
Bottom round/ eye round	1–1½ inches	2–3 hours
Arm roast (boneless)	2 x 2 x 4 inches	1½–2½ hours
Blade roast	2½–3½ pounds	2½–3½ hours
Chuck roast (boneless)	3½–5 pounds	3½–4½ hours
Brisket (fresh)	1–1½ inches	2–3 hours
Round Steak	2 x 2 x 4 inches	1½–2½ hours

Fail-Proof Grilling Method for Beef

Season your steaks with preferred herbs and spices. I Love Montreal steak seasoning; however, it's tough to beat simple coarse grind salt and pepper. Preheat your grill to medium high heat and clean with a wire brush before grilling. Check the time and place steaks on the hot grill. Close the lid for the first 5 minutes of cooking or until droplets of blood appear on the top of the steak. Your meat has now reached 110 degrees. Flip the steak and continue to time the total cooking time per the following chart. Verify doneness using a meat thermometer and take the steaks off the grill when they reach a temperature 5 degrees lower than desired doneness. Your steaks will continue to cook while resting. Let steaks rest on counter for 5-8 minutes before cutting.

Grilling Chart for Steaks

		MINUTES		
TYPE OF STEAK	THICKNESS OR WEIGHT	RARE (140°F)	MEDIUM (160°F)	WELL (170°F)
Rib eye	¾ inch	5–7	7–9	9–11
New York strip	1 inch	8–10	10–12	12–14
Flank steak	1–1½ pounds	10–15	15–19	19–22
Porterhouse, rib, rib eye, sirloin, T-bone, tenderloin, top loin, London broil	1 inch 1½ inches 2 inches	6–7 10–12 15–17	7–9 12–15 17–19	9–11 15–19 19–22

Pork

I love pork! Back ribs, roasts, boneless chops, bone-in chops, country ribs—oh, how the savory dishes abound! ☺ Whether it's a backyard BBQ featuring ribs and loin or a crown roast for a special holiday, pork is sure to please.

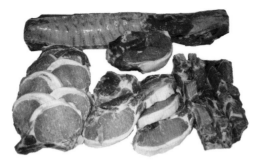

Loin Roast   Crown Roast

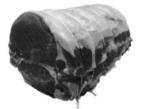 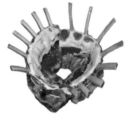

Shoulder Roast from which comes Shoulder Steaks

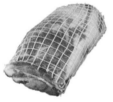 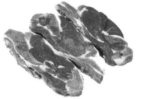

Boston Butt   Rolled Roast

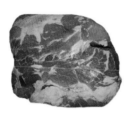 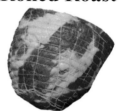

Country Ribs   Ham

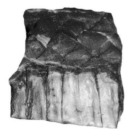 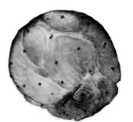

As with the beef roasts, you can see from the pictures there is a major difference in fat content in these roasts. The roast with the least "marbling" is the loin roast. The roast with the most marbling is the Boston butt.

Like beef roasts, some are great for roasting and some are great for braising. Let's discuss the roasts individually.

You'll find the Boston butt a wonderful roast to braise. Cooked slowly with a bit of liquid in a tightly lidded pot or roasting bag, the marbling makes the meat more tender. The fat simply melts away during cooking, leaving gaps in the meat. The end result is a very tender roast perfect for pulled pork.

The loin, on the other hand, has very little fat and needs to be cooked to 140 degrees then removed from heat and allowed to rest for 15 minutes. This roast will supply you with wonderful sliced pork, juicy and full of flavor. Be forewarned, however: cooking this roast beyond 140 degrees will result in a dry roast that requires lots of gravy to make it palatable.

Again, I suggest you buy a good meat thermometer; they are not expensive and they will keep you out of trouble. About three-quarters of the way through the cooking time, check your meat's internal temperature by sticking the thermometer into the center of the roast away from bone. Ovens vary in temperature, so it's a good idea to keep an eye on it.

Once the roast has reached the proper temperature, remove

it from the oven and **let stand 15 to 20 minutes** prior to carving. Letting the roast stand prevents the juices from running out of the roast, which would leave it dry.

Crown roasts are beautiful on the table and offer you wonderful bone-in chops when sliced.

Country ribs are great roasted, grilled, braised, or cut into chunks, trimmed, pan-fried, and slow-cooked in tomato sauce.

Rolled roasts, shoulder, and butt can be roasted or braised. If roasting, cook to well done in order to void the fat out of the roast.

Hams are available both raw and precooked. For a precooked ham, you simply stick several cloves in the ham and place it on a roasting rack in a roasting pan. Pour a cup of water in the bottom of the roasting pan for easy cleanup, preheat your oven to 350 degrees, and bake. An average 5 to 7 pound ham will be heated through in about 45 minutes to 1 hour. Avoid overcooking, as this will result in a dry ham.

Loin roasts are excellent and one of my favorites. I find them on sale all the time for very affordable prices and they offer you options. Loin roasts can be cooked as a whole roast, cut into chops, feathered-stuffed-rolled and roasted, or even cut into chunks for kabobs or stir-fries. I like to buy a loin big enough to give me a variety of everything mentioned above. The meat freezes well, and having it pre-cut makes my job in the kitchen easier.

As with beef, roasting pork works better with some cuts than others. More tender cuts of meat return much better results when dry-roasted. For best results, dry-roast methods (on a rack in a roasting pan) should be limited to the cuts listed in the following chart under ROASTING.

Employ the cooking methods prescribed in my chart for other cuts. Stovetop or grill cooking, braising, stewing, and broiling are all easy cooking methods and will give you good results.

Don't forget braising: this easy technique involves cooking at a low temp in a pot with a tight-fitting lid and a small amount of liquid. Just as when I braise beef, I like to make my life easy when braising pork roasts. I buy an oven-safe roasting bag from the market, place my seasoned roast in it, pour in ½ to ¾ cup of broth, and plop it in the oven for the prescribed time. When the roast is done, the roast and gravy are removed and the bag gets tossed . . . no fuss . . . no muss. ☺

Fail-Proof Dry-Roast Method for Pork

Season the roast with your preferred herbs and spices. Place the roast, fat side up, on a rack in a shallow roasting pan, uncovered, in a 350-degree oven (too tall a pan will result in insufficient browning). Stick an oven-safe meat thermometer into the thickest part of the meat. Be sure to stop in the middle and to avoid the bone. Do not add water; do not cover. Roast the meat until 5 degrees below your desired doneness, then remove from the oven. The pork will continue to cook for the next 10 to 15 minutes on your counter. This will result in the desired finished doneness. Let the roast stand 20 minutes before slicing. This allows the juices to coagulate and avoids a dry roast.

Roasting Chart for Pork

Set the oven to 350 degrees. The meat thermometer should read 140 degrees for rare, 160 degrees for medium, and 170 degrees for well done.

CUT	WEIGHT IN POUNDS	COOKING TIME
Loin roast, bone-in or boneless	2–5	20–30 minutes per pound
Crown roast	4–6	20–30 minutes per pound
Leg (fresh ham) whole, bone-in	12–16	22–26 minutes per pound
Leg (fresh ham) half, bone-in	5–8	35–40 minutes per pound
Boston butt, shoulder, and rolled roasts	3–6	45 minutes per pound
Tenderloin (roast at 425–450°F)	½–1½	20–30 minutes total
Ribs (back, country-style, or spare)	2–4	1½–2 hours (or until fork-tender)

Broiling and Grilling Chart for Pork

Broil 4 inches from the heat source, or cook directly on the grill.

CUT	THICKNESS OR WEIGHT	COOKING TIME
Loin chops, bone-in or boneless	¾ inches 1½ inches	6–8 minutes 12–16 minutes
Tenderloin	½–1½ pounds	15–25 minutes
Ribs, all types (indirect heat)	2–4 pounds	1½–2 hours
Ground pork patties (direct heat)	½ inch	8–10 minutes

Chart for Skillet-Cooking Pork on the Stovetop or Grill

CUT	THICKNESS OR WEIGHT	COOKING TIME
Loin chops or cutlets	¼ inch ¾ inch	3–4 minutes 7–8 minutes
Tenderloin medallions	¼–½ inch	4–8 minutes
Ground pork patties	½ inch	8–10 minutes

Fail-Proof Braising Method for Pork

Season a pork roast with your preferred herbs and spices. Place the roast, fat side up, in a store-bought roasting bag or a Dutch oven with a tight-fitting lid.

Pour in ½ to ¾ cup chicken or beef broth. Beer, water, boxed onion soup mix (watch the label for carbs), or wine may be used instead. Bake in a roasting bag or a Dutch oven.

Braising Chart for Pork

Cover and simmer with liquid in the oven.

CUT	THICKNESS OR WEIGHT	COOKING TIME
Chops, cutlets, cubes, medallions	Up to 1 inch	10–25 minutes
Boston butt, boneless	3–6 pounds	2–2 ½ hours
Ribs, all types	2–4 pounds	1½–2 hours

Stewing Chart for Pork

Cover the pan and simmer with a liquid on the stovetop.

CUT	THICKNESS OR WEIGHT	COOKING TIME
Ribs, all types	2–4 pounds	2–2½ hours, or until tender
Cubes	1-inch	45–60 minutes

Lamb

Leg   Crown Roast

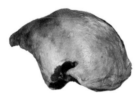 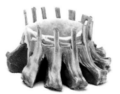

Lamb Rack Roast from which comes Lamb Chops

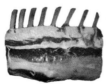 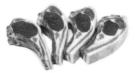

Boneless Shoulder Roast Boneless Leg Roast

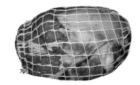 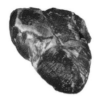

As with beef and pork roasts, you can see from the pictures that lamb comes in various cuts. Lamb is a wonderful, flavorful meat overlooked by many shoppers. Follow the roasting charts below and bring lamb into your kitchen.

Roasting Chart for Lamb

CUT	COOKING TEMPERA-TURE	WEIGHT IN POUNDS	MINUTES PER POUND		
			RARE 140°	MEDIUM 160°	WELL 170°
Whole leg	325°F	5–7	14	22	27
		7–9	18	27	33
Half leg shank	325°F	3–4	23	30	35
Half leg sirloin	325°F	3–4	22	33	43
Crown roast	375°F	2–3	21	28	33
Shoulder roast, boneless	325°F	4–6	32	38	43
Shoulder roast, bone-in	325°F	4–6	18	23	28
Rib roast or rack of ribs	375°F	1½–2½	28	32	38

Poultry

Duck   Goose

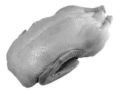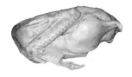

Turkey Boneless Turkey Roast

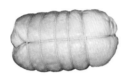

Chicken Rock Cornish Hens

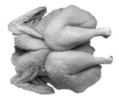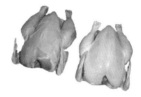

Have you ever had a roasted Rock Cornish hen? They're wonderful! It's like eating your own little "mini me" chicken. You get to enjoy all the parts of your hen without having to share the breasts, drumsticks, wings, or thighs. How about a boneless turkey roast? Slice into it and see the magic of white meat and dark meat in the same slice. Step outside the chicken box and explore the wonderful world of poultry.

As my kids used to say:
Duck Duck Goose

Cooking Charts for Poultry

It's important to cook poultry thoroughly. Red or pink juices should never be present when serving. The following charts are meant to be used as guidelines. Always check poultry cooking progression with a meat thermometer.

Roasting Chart for Poultry

Poultry should be fully thawed and at room temperature when it is placed in the oven.

TYPE OR CUT OF POULTRY	TEMPERA-TURE	WEIGHT IN POUNDS	COOKING TIME, UNSTUFFED
Chicken, whole roaster	350°F	2½–3	1¼–1½ hours
		3–4	1½–1¾ hours
		4–6	1¾–2 hours
Rock Cornish hen	350°F	1–2	1–1¼ hours
Capon	325°F	5–6	1¾–2 hours
		6–8	2¼–3½ hours
Turkey, whole	325°F	8–12	2¾–3 hours
		12–14	3–3¾ hours
		14–18	3¾–4¼ hours
		18–20	4¼–4½ hours
		20–24	4½–5 hours

TYPE OR CUT OF POULTRY	TEMPERA-TURE	WEIGHT IN POUNDS	COOKING TIME, UNSTUFFED
Turkey, cut-up	325°F	2–3	50–60 minutes
Breast, half		4–6	1½–2¼hours
Breast, whole		6–8	2¼–3¼ hours
Breast, whole		¾–1	2–2¼ hours
Drumsticks		¾–1	1¾–2 hours
Thighs		6–8	1¾–2¼ hours
Wings			
Goose	350°F	10–12	2¾–3¼ hours
Duck	350°F	4–5	2–2½ hours

Stewing Chart for Poultry

This chart is for poultry cooked in liquid in a covered pot on the stove.

TYPE OR CUT OF POULTRY	WEIGHT	COOKING TIME
Whole broiler or fryer	3–4 pounds	1–1¼ hours
Whole roaster	5–7 pounds	1¾–2 hours
Whole Cornish hens	18–24 ounces	35–40 minutes
Breast half, bone-in	6–8 ounces	35–45 minutes
Breast half, boneless	4 ounces	25–30 minutes
Leg or thigh	8 or 4 ounces	40–50 minutes
Drumstick	4 ounces	40–50 minutes
Wing or wingette/drumette	2–3 ounces	35–45 minutes

Grilling Chart for Poultry

This chart is for poultry cooked on the grill over **indirect** heat.

TYPE OR CUT OF POULTRY	WEIGHT	COOKING TIME, UNSTUFFED
Whole broiler or fryer	3–4 pounds	60–70 minutes
Whole roaster	5–7 pounds	18–25 minutes/pound
Whole Cornish hens	18–24 ounces	45–55 minutes
Whole turkey	8–12 pounds	2–3 hours
	12–16 pounds	3–4 hours
Whole duck	4½ pounds	2½ hours
Whole goose	8–12 pounds	18–20 minutes/pound
Whole capon	4–8 pounds	15–20 minutes/pound
Breast half, bone-in	6–8 ounces	10–15 minutes/side
Breast half, boneless	4 ounces	8–10 minutes/side
	6–8 ounces	10–15 minutes/side
Leg or thigh	8 or 4 ounces	10–15 minutes/side
Drumstick	4 ounces	8–12 minutes/side
	8–16 ounces	10–15 minutes/side
Wing or wingette/drumette	2–3 ounces	8–12 minutes/side

Braising Chart for Poultry

This chart is for cooking poultry in an oven bag at 350 degrees.

TYPE OR CUT OF POULTRY	WEIGHT IN POUNDS	COOKING TIME, UNSTUFFED
Whole turkey	8–12	1½–2 hours
	12–16	2–2½ hours
	16–20	2½–3 hours
	20–24	3–3½ hours

TYPE OR CUT OF POULTRY	WEIGHT IN POUNDS	COOKING TIME, UNSTUFFED
Turkey breast, bone-in	4–8	1¼–2 hours
	10–12	2¼–2¾ hours
Turkey breast, boneless	2½–3	1¼–1¾ hours
	5–7	2–2 ¾ hours
	8–12	3–3½ hours
Turkey drumsticks	1–3	1½–1¾ hours
Chicken pieces	2–3	45–50 minutes
Chicken thighs	½–2¼	35–40 minutes
Chicken drumsticks	1–2½	35–40 minutes
Chicken breast half, bone-in	1–2½	40–45 minutes
Chicken Breast half, boneless	¾–1½	25–30 minutes
Whole chicken	3½–4	1–1¼ hours
	5–7	1¼–1½ hours
Cornish hens	1½–3½	40–45 minutes
	4–7	55–60 minutes

How to Choose the Right Spice

Herb/Spice	Flavor	Use	Use In
Allspice	Clove/cinnamon	Ground	Squash, pumpkin,
Anise	Licorice	Ground	Cooked spinach, fish, poultry
Basil	Italian	Fresh	Tomatoes, eggplant, salad, pasta, pizza, pork, fish, omelets
Bay leaf	Pine	Dried whole leaves	Soups, stews sauces, seafood boils, beans
Black peppercorns	Semi-hot	Dried, freshly ground	Any dish requiring mild heat
White peppercorns	Hot	Dried, freshly ground	Any dish requiring medium heat; mix with other peppercorns in grinder
Green peppercorns	Bitter	Dried, freshly ground	Mix with other peppercorns in grinder
Red peppercorns	Sweet	Dried, freshly ground	Mix with other peppercorns in grinder
Capers	Pickled	In brine	Salads, eggs, salmon
Caraway	Rye	Whole seeds	Sausage
Cardamom	Mild, sweet, spicy, strong	Whole or ground	Stews, soups
Cayenne pepper	Very hot	Dried flakes or ground	Any dish requiring extreme heat
Celery seed	Celery	Dried whole seed	Cole slaw, salads, soups, sauces
Chervil	Parsley	Freshly chopped	Casseroles, salads, soups, egg dishes, Italian dishes
Chili powder	Spicy, earthy, medium heat	Ground	Southwestern dishes

Herb/Spice	Flavor	Use	Use In
Chives	Onion/garlic	Freshly chopped	Egg dishes, cheese balls, salads
Cilantro	Mild bittersweet	Freshly chopped	Salsas, pico de gallo, southwestern dishes
Cinnamon	Strong bittersweet	Sticks or ground	Middle Eastern dishes, coffee, squash, ham
Cloves	Strong bittersweet	Whole or ground	Ham, corned beef, roast poultry, roasted onions, stews, curries
Coriander	Spicy/sweet, sometimes hot	Ground or whole	Pickling spice (mix with mustard seed), corned beef
Cumin	Peppery	Ground	Southwestern and Mexican dishes
Curry powder	Hot/strong	Ground, add in small amounts	Curries
Dill	Pickley, aromatic	Freshly chopped or seeds	Fish dishes, sauces, dips, egg dishes
Fennel	Light licorice	Raw or cooked	Roasted bulb, raw in salads, cooked in stews
Garlic	Strong/spicy/ hot/aromatic	Freshly chopped, roasted	Italian dishes, sauces, roasted, stews, soups, meat rubs, salads, sea-food sautés, marinades
Ginger	Spicy/hot	Freshly grated or dried powder	Asian dishes, stir-fries
Horseradish	Hot	Creamed	Roast beef condiment, seafood sauce (mixed with sugar-free ketchup)

Herb/Spice	Flavor	Use	Use In
Mace	Strong nutmeg	Ground	Meatloaf, meatballs, baked fish, cabbage, stir-fries
Marjoram	Very mild	Fresh or dried	Soups, seafood, egg dishes
Mint	Strong/minty/cool	Fresh	Salads, vegetable dishes, coffee
Mustard seed	Strong/slight bitter/tangy/hot	Whole seed	Pickling spice (mixed with coriander), corned beef
Nutmeg	Aromatic, spicy/sweet	Freshly ground	Coffee, stir-fries, egg dishes, pot roasts, meatloaf, meatballs
Oregano	Italian	Fresh or dried	Italian dishes, soups, pizza, tomato sauces, chili
Paprika	Sweet/colorful	Ground powder	Hungarian dishes, garnish on deviled eggs
Parsley	Mild/fresh/clean	Fresh	Italian dishes, egg dishes, garnish, marinades, roast rubs, soups, salads
Poppy seed	Nutty	Dried, whole	Salad dressings, salads, sauces, stir-fries
Rosemary	Strong aromatic, pine	Fresh	Lamb roasts, baked salmon, fish dishes
Saffron	Colorful	Dried	Coloring element for sauces, Middle Eastern dishes, Indian dishes
Sage	Earthy	Fresh or dried	Poultry, sausage
Sesame seed	Nutty	Whole black and white	Stir-fries, marinades, salads, coating on tuna steaks, Asian dishes, Korean ribs, salad dressing

Herb/Spice	Flavor	Use	Use In
Tarragon	Licorice	Fresh	Flavored vinegars, vegetable stir-fries, egg dishes, fish dishes, sauces, salads
Thyme	Minty, lemony	Fresh or dried	Roasts, poultry
Turmeric	Colorful	Ground	Curries, Middle Eastern and Indian dishes, coloring for sauces
Vanilla	Aromatic/sweet	Extract	Cheesecake, coffee

WEIGHTS AND MEASUREMENTS

Common Measurements	
1 tablespoon (T) =	3 teaspoons (tsp)
$\frac{1}{16}$ cup =	1 tablespoon
$\frac{1}{8}$ cup =	2 tablespoons
$\frac{1}{6}$ cup =	2 tablespoons + 2 teaspoons
$\frac{1}{4}$ cup =	4 tablespoons
$\frac{1}{3}$ cup =	5 tablespoons + 1 teaspoon
$\frac{3}{8}$ cup =	6 tablespoons
$\frac{1}{2}$ cup =	8 tablespoons
$\frac{2}{3}$ cup =	10 tablespoons + 2 teaspoons
$\frac{3}{4}$ cup =	12 tablespoons
1 cup =	48 teaspoons
1 cup =	16 tablespoons
8 fluid ounces (fl ounces) =	1 cup
1 pint (pt) =	2 cups
1 quart (qt) =	2 pints
4 cups =	1 quart
1 gallon (gal) =	4 quarts

U.S. Measurements to Metric System			
Size		Weight	
⅕ teaspoon =	1 milliliter	1 ounce =	28 grams
1 teaspoon =	5 ml	1 pound =	454 grams
1 tablespoon =	15 ml		
1 fluid ounce =	30 ml		
⅕ cup =	47 ml		
1 cup =	237 ml		
2 cups = 1 pint =	473 ml		
4 cups = 1 quart =	.95 liter		
4 quarts = 1 gal =	3.8 liters		

Metric Measure to US			
Size		Weight	
1 milliliter =	⅕ teaspoon	1 gram =	.035 ounce
5 ml =	1 teaspoon	100 grams =	3.5 ounces
15 ml =	1 tablespoon	500 grams =	1.10 pounds
100 ml =	3.4 fluid ounces	1 kilogram =	2.205 pounds 35 ounces
240 ml =	1 cup		
1 liter =	34 fluid ounces 4.2 cups 2.1 pints 1.06 quarts 0.26 gallon		

FAT TO SKINNY PORTION SIZES AT A GLANCE

Common Equivalents	
Fruits and Veggies	
1 cup chopped fruit =	A baseball
1 cup chopped salad =	A baseball
½ cup cooked veggies =	A tennis ball
Meat and Poultry	
3 ounces =	A deck of cards
8 ounces =	A small paperback book
Fish, Cheese and Nuts	
3 ounces fish =	A checkbook
1 ounce cheese =	4 dice
1 ounce nuts =	2 ping-pong balls

EPILOGUE

Thank you for taking the time to allow me to share my story with you. I wrote **FAT TO SKINNY Fast and Easy!** because I knew I could help people of all ages. There's simply no reason for anyone to go through life as a **FAT** person if they know the secrets. With the rising obesity problem our nation is facing, children's education became an important part of my mission. I tried to write this book to be easily understood by all ages, and if you have children I urge you to have them read it. Starting your kids eating right when they are young will be a lifelong gift they will appreciate as they get older. Before you start your program, take a BEFORE photo of yourself and email it to me. I'll be rooting for you and will look forward to your AFTER photo showing your success. I would like to hear from you and learn how the information contained in this book has helped to change your life. Please feel free to contact me by email:

dougvarrieur@fattoskinny.com

GENERAL INDEX

INDEX OF RECIPES AND INGREDIENTS

ABOUT THE AUTHOR

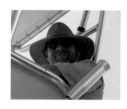

Doug Varrieur

Entrepreneur, businessman, father, stepfather, husband, ex-husband, son, stepson, partner, ex-partner, writer, and philosopher

Here are some interesting facts about the author. When Doug wrote **FAT TO SKINNY Fast and Easy!**, he was 50 years young. He had battled weight gain his entire life until he found the secrets. Being **FAT** never held him back, and over the past 27 years he built and sold 3 successful companies and worked extensively as a business consultant. The only challenge Doug couldn't succeed at over the years was weight control. He put all of his effort and time into finding the secrets to **FAT** loss and good health. He succeeded, quickly and easily losing over 100 pounds with his own methods. Next came Sherri's amazing 70-pound **FAT** loss, all without diets, surgery, drugs, or exercise. Doug found the SECRET! **FAT TO SKINNY Fast and Easy!** was written because he wanted to share his secrets with the world. Years after this amazing weight loss, Doug and Sherri, his beautiful wife, continue to enjoy being thin and healthy. They concentrate on living a well-balanced and happy life.